a promise kept

HONORING HIS WISHES, EMBRACING OUR LOVE

erica baccus

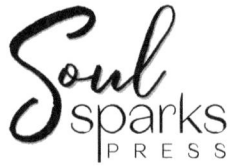

The opinions expressed in this publication are the author's own. This publication is sold with the understanding that the author and publisher are not engaged in rendering psychological, financial, or other professional services. If expert advice or counseling is needed, the reader is encouraged to consult a professional.

ISBN for Softcover: 979-8-9922748-4-4
ISBN for Hardcover: 979-8-9922748-7-5

Copyright © 2025 Soul Sparks Press. All Rights Reserved. No part of this publication may be reproduced, distributed, or transmitted in any form or by any means, including photocopying, recording, or other electronic or mechanical methods, without the prior written permission of the publisher, except in the case of brief quotations embodied in critical reviews and certain other noncommercial uses permitted by copyright law. For permission requests, please contact the publisher at soulsparkspress.com.

Contents

Prologue	v	Doing It Myself	111
		Vietnam	117
John's Request Letter	1	John's Journey	119
Biographical Statement		Backpacking	127
for John Baccus	5	The Peach Tree	137
Trust Your Lust	9	Love and Frustration	139
How Long is		The Next Pregnancy	145
Five to Six Years?	15	The Move	151
The Day the Music Died	21	Papa John	155
Super Bowl Sunday	27	The Caretaker	159
Courtship	31	Tomatoes	163
What's On My Mind	39	Sharing The News	165
We Were Not a Match	43	2022: A Turning Point	181
Day To Day	49	September 23, 2022	193
The Splits	55	Breakfast Talk	195
Nothing Is Forever	61	The Popcorn Kernel	199
Wedding Bells Rang	77	Trains	203
Family Man	83	Anniversaries	209
Ski Story	87	Measuring	221
Boston	89	Choosing The Date	227
Lox and Bagels	101	The Dentist	233
Days of Our Lives	103	Choosing My Escort	237

Owen's Graduation	241	The Day the Ashes Came	301
The Farewell Tour	247	Journal Notes	303
Traditions	255	Life After	311
Medical Mania	259	Afterword	315
Our Last Night	263	What's It All About, Alfie?	317
John's Wallet	267	Grieving	321
Hotel Boldern	271	Things I Wish	
The Flight Home	283	I Could Ask John	327
The Unexpected Overnight	287		
The Sunroom	291	*Appendix*	329
Good-bye Letter	293	*Acknowledgements*	351
Planning The Memorial	295		

Prologue

I sat in the impersonal, well furnished, sterile waiting room once a week waiting for the stroke of 10 AM. On time, every time, my therapist walked in holding a notebook in her hand. She nodded at me. I stood, smiled and said, "Good morning."

I followed her into her office, where she allowed me to choose the sofa or the chair. "How are you, Erica?"

"I'm fine, thank you." Our relationship was polite. We were polite strangers attempting to discuss the most serious and difficult issues.

When we first met, I had told her why I was seeking help. "I don't need to change who I am. I do not need help with any personal problems. I am here because my husband has Alzheimer's, and he is declining. I do not know how to feel. I do not know how to live each day in my terror. I need someone to listen to me. I need someone to hear me. I am holding my thoughts and feelings inside with no way to express them."

She replied, "I understand. I am not an expert on Alzheimer's, but I am sure I can help you through this difficult time."

We moved to Zoom after a while just because it was easier. Each week, the script was the same. I'd describe a new symptom that John displayed, which added stress to each already stressful day. She listened to me talk about my sadness and feelings of loss and confusion, but she seemed unable to grasp the depth of my fears. I kept waiting for her to say something—do something—that would lessen my fears.

I needed someone to help me navigate the waters of despair as John's illness progressed. I needed someone to listen to my darkest thoughts—someone who could listen without feeling the need to "cure" me nor judge me. However, she seemed incapable of understanding the whole encompassing nightmare we were living through.

I think, out of desperation on her part, she recommended that I read a book she heard about. "Erica," she said, "I heard there is a book for people who are struggling with Alzheimer's. I haven't read it yet, but it is supposed to be helpful for caretakers as well as the afflicted person." To this day I believe she had no idea of the role she played in how John and I ended his life with Alzheimer's.

By some sort of fate, my therapist recommended I read a book written by a famous novelist who is also a psychotherapist who just happened to write the exact book about what I was trying to understand. She unwittingly became an important person in our saga.

It is called *In Love* by Amy Bloom.

I knew who Amy Bloom was. I knew she was an award-winning novelist. But I had not heard of *In Love*. So, on May 4, 2022, I bought the book on Amazon. I read it in two days. I reread it again a few months later to take notes and underline necessary points. I tried talking to my therapist about the book in future meetings, but she never found the time to read it. Ultimately, I discontinued my relationship with my therapist because she could not discuss *In Love* with me. I felt frustrated that she did not seem to understand how seriously I needed help. Was it not worth her time to read a book she recommended to me that might have shed some light on the distress my husband and I were experiencing?

Amy Bloom's story detailed how she helped her husband die. He had Alzheimer's and did not want to live through the painful disease just as John did not want to experience this kind of suffering. Amy Bloom conducted her own research and found one of the only two places in the world one can turn to for an accompanied suicide for people who have dementia: Dignitas in Zurich, Switzerland. I saw her book as a "how-to" manual on ending your life peacefully, painlessly, and with dignity.

Amy's book was a road map for me at a time when I could not find my way out of the morass. I shall always be grateful to Amy Bloom for sharing her story so we could follow in her footsteps. She showed me the way out of our confusion and John's fear of having to die in a vegetative state. She showed me her courage which I needed to emulate. She demonstrated that it was possible to help your husband die and you would survive.

I had no intention of writing our story. However, after John died, when I was a complete zombie and unable to sort out my feelings, I realized Amy Bloom's book was only part of it. I felt compelled to write about our experience from a different perspective. Writing was part of my healing process, partly to answer the questions so many have asked me and partly to help understand what had just happened to our lives. I needed to write about the emotional distress John and I experienced throughout his illness and the end of life. I needed to write about the joy we shared even through the worst of days. I needed to express it all in context of our magical marriage we had for forty-one years.

Perhaps, one day someone will think of *A Promise Kept* as a path to understanding their own similar trauma.

John's Request Letter

January 30, 2023

Dear Sir,

I am writing to you today to formally request Dignitas to prepare an accompanied suicide for me. I am currently suffering from Alzheimer's. I was diagnosed in January 2020 and the illness is progressing. I am still functional, but I do not want to live through the end stages of this disease, which would incapacitate me both physically and mentally. I believe the process of living requires an awareness that Alzheimer's will eventually take away from me. In light of that, planning and executing my death prior to those devastating aspects of my disease allows me to die with dignity, but more importantly, not live with the inability to be the master of my own life. This decision is not lightly taken.

How is it that John could write so eloquently? I do believe John was very clear about his decision. This should help me accept it.

I am physically in good health, except for Alzheimer's and its associated symptoms. I am suffering from Myoclonus, which causes me to shake internally and externally constantly. I am losing energy quickly in addition to the loss of my short-term memory. On occasion I have lapses where my reality is not grounded in fact.

My short-term memory loss is increasing at a relatively rapid rate. I don't know the day of the week or the date. I can't remember to go to places where I am supposed to be. I am told I ask the same questions repeatedly and tell the same stories over and over.

I had to help John remember how he was declining—what the specifics were.

I spend many of my days sitting in a chair watching TV or sleeping, which is a huge change from what was normal. I used to work in the garden each day or work on building my train in the garage, ride a bike or go for a hike. I no longer have the energy to do any of those activities which I loved.

I dress myself, shower and overall can take care of my bodily needs. However, I no longer can pay our bills, remember to fix the needed repairs in our tenants' homes, or take care of our overall financial requirements.

My diagnosis and the progression of my disease have all brought me to the conclusion that my life will be considerably less viable in a relatively short period of time. I believe in life. I believe in the dignity of life and I truly believe life is not something to be wasted.

It hurt to watch John compose this. I had to type it for him. It was one of the steps in the process that had to be completed and approved. Surreal was a word I used over and over to myself.

Erica Baccus

I am happy to answer any questions you may have.

Respectfully,

John Baccus

Biographical Statement for John Baccus

I was born on November 16, 1945, in Burbank, CA. Less than a year after my birth, my parents separated and my mother and my three older siblings and I moved to a small rural community in Southern California called Lake Elsinore. Early in my youth, the lake lost its water rights and eventually dried up, thus making the area pretty impoverished. My mom was on welfare (aid to dependent children) my entire childhood. In spite of not having a lot of money, I had a full and enjoyable childhood. The rural nature of Elsinore allowed my siblings and me to build forts together, sleep outside in the summer, hike, bike, and generally have a lot of fun outside.

I attended school in Elsinore from kindergarten through high school and always was an excellent student. In my senior year of high school, my principal helped me get a scholarship to college. He explained that his wife was attending California State College at Fullerton, which was about 40 miles from Elsinore. He volunteered that she would drive me to and from school each day. He then handed me an application to this college and told me to fill it out. I was accepted to Cal State Fullerton and fortunately received partial scholarships. This simple act of kindness changed the direction of my life.

I eventually moved to Fullerton, CA to be closer to school. Because the scholarships could not cover all my expenses, I had to supplement my income by working while attending school. I worked for Hunt Wesson Foods (a cannery) on swing shifts which are from 3 PM to 11 PM. Classes started around 8 AM. For the most part the shifts in the cannery were 8 hours long, however, there were times when the job required me to work 12-hour shifts which made it impossible for me to stay in school.

I dropped out of school in 1966 and was immediately drafted into the US Army and eventually served in Vietnam. Luckily I was able to get an early release from the Army after 21 months to return to college. I finished school on the GI Bill with a degree in Business. (The U.S. government paid veterans a stipend to attend college.)

I have always been drawn to the manufacturing process— I have loved building things—and enjoyed a career in manufacturing management. I worked mostly in the medical diagnostic industry until I founded my own company, Baccus Machinery, in 1982.

In 1972, I married my first wife. We had one son together, Kyle, and she had a daughter, Lori, from another marriage. We moved to the SF Bay Area to be closer to family in 1976. Both Kyle and Lori are very close to me even though my wife and I separated in 1979.

Erica and I met at work and we became good friends. Eventually, we fell in love and married in 1982. She had a son from a previous marriage who was 14 when we married and he and I grew into close friends. We have had a glorious, full, loving marriage for 40 years. We now have 5 grandchildren- three from my son and two from Erica's son. We are a loving, happy, blended family and love to all spend time together.

Erica Baccus

We have lived in San Francisco, CA since 1993 and have both retired. We love our city and all that it offers. We have spent the last 40 years camping, backpacking, skiing, biking, hiking, playing golf, and enjoying the wonderful outdoors living in California affords us. We have taken family trips with our kids and grandkids. We have traveled all over the world throughout our marriage including Europe, Africa, Australia and New Zealand. We have had a fortunate and lovely life. Of course, now things have changed and I can no longer do much of what I had enjoyed doing when I was healthy.

Erica is supporting me completely in my desire to have a self-determined end of life and she will be the person accompanying me to Switzerland. We have been making decisions together for 40 years and this is the most difficult one of our lives, but we are in total agreement.

Respectfully,

John Baccus

Trust Your Lust

I met John on my first day of work at SmithKline Diagnostics on a February day in 1977. I had a brand new job as a customer service executive for the diagnostics department. I joined a group of about 10 women who sat in one large room with computer printouts, which identified which customers were having a problem with their orders. I was given a territory and told to figure out how to solve customers' problems.

Before I even sat down to work on that very first day, I met John. I was standing in the large lobby area in front of our office space talking to my new boss, Dorothy. In the middle of our conversation, a tall, handsome man dressed in navy blue pants and a white shirt unbuttoned at the top and loose tie strolled up to Dorothy for some work-related question. He was polite and seemed unusually at ease and friendly. Dorothy introduced us. John was 31; I was 33.

"Erica, this is John Baccus. He's the manufacturing manager here and is responsible for packaging our product. John, this is Erica. It's her first day at work. She'll be reporting to me."

"Nice to meet you, Erica. Congratulations on your new job! Has anyone given you a tour of the building yet?"

"No." I looked at Dorothy for permission and she nodded her head to say *go with him.*

SmithKline was a very lengthy building with manufacturing at the back and marketing/sales in the front. John was a manufacturing manager in charge of packaging and my new job was located in the marketing area.

"Welcome, Erica. I'll introduce you to some people you will need to know. It's a very friendly place here, so feel free to stop by and talk to anyone."

"Thanks, John. This is very nice of you to take time out for me." We stopped by an office where the door was open.

"Hi Martha," John said. "This is Erica. It's her first day here. I know you two will get to know each other. Erica, this is Martha. She is head of Human Resources and a very funny lady."

The usual nice–to–meet–yous were exchanged, and we went on.

"Hey, Richard, meet Erica. She is working for Dorothy in customer service. First day today. I bet you are going to be a big help to her."

"Hi Erica, welcome aboard. If you need help understanding the chemistry in our products, I love to teach."

"Thanks a lot. I will definitely remember you said that."

John kept strolling to the back of the building introducing me to Margaret, Ed, Ron and his own boss, Les, until we reached his office.

"This is my sanctuary away from the crowds. Have a seat for a minute and then I'll walk you back."

I watched John push aside a pile of papers and light a cigarette pulling an already overflowing ashtray closer to him. Then I saw the surprise.

Behind John's chair was a magnificent aquarium filled with multi-colored tropical fish. I thought *what a strange thing to have in an office.* "John, that is a beautiful aquarium. I guess you are fond of fish?"

"Ya, I really like to sit back, have a toke on my joint and watch the fish swim. It relaxes me."

I went to sleep at night thinking about my day at work and felt content. Perhaps this was the place I could call home for a while. This would be the company that would be my new beginning. I could stop worrying about how I would pay the rent and earn enough to buy Christmas presents for Danny and feel good about myself.

It had been hard to leave teaching and find a fulfilling job to support myself and Danny. I had several jobs before this one which were short-lived for one reason or another. I was getting frustrated and a bit frightened that I may never find my place. I had high hopes this company would be my answer. My first day felt promising. People were friendly, yet professional. I caught on to the job quickly and Dorothy, my boss, was very kind.

I thought, "I think I'll like this job."

That night-that first night-I dreamed of John in his navy blue pants and sexy long legs and beautiful blue eyes. I woke up in the morning, stood by the side of my bed thinking about my dream and said to myself,

"No, Erica, you can't dream about him. He is married and you are living with someone." I thought, "Well, I can't help what I dream about," but I was unconvincing.

John and I built a friendship through our work. I had a lot of contact with him as I moved into a new job working for Carol, who was responsible for custom-packaged products. I started working for her as a side job to my real position in customer service. It was a way to work my way up the ladder. It took about six months for me to get a full-time job with Carol. I had to get custom diagnostic tests created, packaged and sent out to specific customers. John, of course, was the packaging manager. So, I had a lot of long walks down that long hallway to talk to John about my projects. He was always friendly—always with a smile and a warm greeting. I could hear his familiar, full hearty laugh all the way down the hallway.

Over the next few years, I realized I needed to break up with my boyfriend who was living with me. Bob and I were in that phase of a relationship where we irritated each other, we nitpicked the little things and were generally behaving more like strangers than anyone in a romantic relationship. It was past the time of calling it quits, but it seemed harder to do than to just keep the status quo.

I discussed Bob with John continuously. John used to say, "Come to my office and we will discuss it." Then he took me outside to the curb where he smoked a cigarette and maybe I did too and we discussed my romantic problems. I could always count on John to listen. He never ever told me to break up—he just listened. Somewhere along the way, I was falling in love with John.

Conversations about Bob went something like this:

Erica: "John, I just don't want to be with him anymore. I am not in love with him."

John: "Erica, you should talk with Bob. You will need to figure this out sooner or later."

Erica: " Ugh, I know. I just hate the idea of hurting his feelings."

John: "Is it a good idea to live with someone you don't love because you don't want to hurt his feelings? Maybe if you talk with him, you will be able to work something out."

Erica: "I don't want to work something out."

How Long is Five to Six Years?

I realize the doctors estimate from the time one is diagnosed, but both John and I worried about his memory as early as 2017. He went undiagnosed-formally-for three more years, but looking back now I do believe we fit right into the average.

The summer of 2017, Owen, our first grandchild, turned thirteen and Noah, our number-two grandson, would be eleven in October. We took the boys camping in Big Trees in Arnold, California with Kiera and Taryn, (friends the same age as the boys) and then we joined the annual California family reunion in Tahoe which we all loved. In September, John and I traveled to Europe.

This was the year we decided not to go to Africa, but to see parts of Europe we had not yet visited: Poland, Prague, Vienna, and Hungary. It really turned out to be a "roots" trip for me, spending time with Ted and Agata (our nephew and niece) in their home in Poland, visiting my mom's home and the birth of her romance with dad in Vienna and Budapest. It was all fun, so very historically interesting-beautiful and at times highly emotional.

One day as we were trying to return to our hotel in Vienna, I noticed John with the map in his hands and behaving rather confused. Yes, he still wanted to use a paper map. I was the more technology-centered advocate in our union. John was and had always been a notoriously gifted map reader. I have always been in awe because I can't read a map. I asked, "What's wrong, John? Are you having a problem? Can I help?" No answer. He just kept turning the map around ninety degrees at a time. The more I asked, the more agitated he became. Finally, I realized we were getting nowhere fast so I took out my iPhone and asked for directions to our place.

John was angry. "Why did you do that? The situation was turning into an argument which I didn't really want to have and really had no idea why we were having it. I guess I was hurting his pride.

The whole event stirred up doubts about what was happening to John, but I tucked it away. Certainly, vacation was not the place to be thinking scary thoughts. I needed to put these thoughts away for a while.

I also started to notice that each day John asked me in an anxious voice, "What are we doing today? Where are we going? Do we have a guide today? How long will we be gone?" This was strange because I always prepped him the day before, but I tossed it to the back of my mind.

When we returned home, everything with John was totally normal. He was his same old confident and capable self. I chalked the mishaps up to thinking he was just uncomfortable in a strange environment. I said nothing to him or anyone else. I put the whole issue out of mind where I wanted it to stay forever.

I was good at this denial thing. I wanted to stay happy. And, besides, John seemed okay, so it wasn't that hard to reside in my own reality. It occupied a space in the back of my brain, ignorable yet there.

As time passed, John often complained to me he was forgetting things. "Erica, there is something wrong with me. I can't remember things I should."

I consoled him and myself with, "I forget things too. Everyone I know at our age forgets things. I can't remember a movie I saw a week ago."

John sometimes countered with, "But this is different." I worried a little bit, but mostly I thought John was exaggerating or just overly concerned. Denial was the most comfortable place.

Weeks and months passed. Sometime, probably in 2018 or early 2019, John mentioned to our primary care doctor that he was concerned about his memory. I was with him at the appointment. We both really liked and respected our primary doctor and he was easy to talk to. The doctor did not make a big deal out of it, but right then and there, he gave John the standard quick memory test. Count backwards from ten, add numbers together, what year is it, name the months backwards and so on. John aced the test.

However, the doctor did suggest to John, "Listen, if you are seriously concerned you can be evaluated by the UCSF Memory Clinic. I'll put a referral and a phone number in your doctors' files for you. You can call them for an appointment." I was relieved. John didn't just ace the test; he answered the questions better and faster than I could. I told myself *we are fine. John is fine.*

John never called. We both let it go until finally in December 2019, I called for an appointment.

I called because I was starting to be concerned. I noticed he was forgetting things he shouldn't: what day it was, or the day or time of his golf date or when he last talked to Kyle.

I talked to my sister, Judy, who is a nurse and who probably knows more about medicine today than many doctors. She lives in Wisconsin, but Judy and I talk on the phone a lot and she is my "person." I confided in her that I was worried about John. She told me, "Erica, if you really are worried, you should take John to a neurologist. They have meds now to slow down Alzheimer's—if he has that—and the earlier you get diagnosed the better."

"I get it, Judy. I need to think about it. I am not sure I will get John to go. But maybe."

"Erica, it's a lot to process. Take your time. Nothing is going to change in a week or a day or a month. But the sooner the better."

"Thanks Judy. Thanks for always being there for me. Bye."

Well maybe the drugs can help if he has Alzheimer's. I can hope.

So, I had a conversation with John telling him what Judy said. John was always so rational about his disease. With his permission, I called UCSF Aging and Memory Center and made the appointment for January.

Now, I had to think about it.

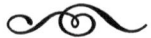

Loving Him

He's losing himself
I'm losing my heart
He's trying so hard
I'm helping him try
He's showing his pain
I feel his futility
He gives me his love
I take all I can get.

The Day the Music Died

It was the morning of January 24, 2020 when John and I drove to the UCSF Memory and Aging Center. It was not a place I looked forward to visiting and I assume John must have been a bit nervous just because of the nature of our appointment.

The office is at the Mission Bay location, a huge, overwhelming facility that always makes me nervous about finding a parking place, finding the right building, being on time and generally just driving there. John drove, and I navigated.

"What time is it," he asked? "Are we running late?" "Who are we meeting with?" We were on time and parked the car easily and found the building with no problem, much to my relief.

We were told to plan a full day of meetings with the doctors for both of us. We were warned some would be with John alone and some with both of us and some with me alone. We were told there was a place for lunch next door where we could escape to between appointments.

We treated the whole thing as routine. We did not become anxious about the tests John had to take or the interviews in which I participated.

The doctors mostly asked me questions to verify John's behavior.

"What kinds of things do you notice John forgets?"

"Well, he has trouble remembering events we have scheduled and what day it is."

"Does he have trouble remembering names of people?"

"No, not really. Actually, he is better at that than I am when we talk about famous people."

"Has he gotten lost?"

"No, he drives himself to golf every week and he drives when we travel together, but sometimes he'll forget where we are going in the middle of the trip."

"Anything else you'd like to add?"

"Well, in 2017 when we were traveling in Europe, all of a sudden, he couldn't read a map, couldn't remember what we did the day before or what I had told him we were going to do today. But, when we got home again, he returned to normal."

John went from one kind of doctor to the other pretty much in his normal good humor, happy to answer questions, talk about himself and draw some clocks on a piece of paper. My participation was minimal, and I provided anecdotal information to corroborate or not corroborate whatever the more objective inquiries were finding.

I was frightened but not willing to say it out loud. I wished and hoped that this—whatever this was—would be fixable. But in the logical part of my brain, I knew something was terribly wrong.

I sat in the waiting room, either waiting for my turn or for John to return from his current meeting. It was like any other doctor's waiting room, but it was dim and quiet. I sat in a chair reading something on my iPhone and was barely able to concentrate. John returned from his first meeting. I asked, "How did it go?"

"Fine, " he said.

"Can you tell me what they asked you? What did you have to do?"

"Well, this felt like a getting-to-know you they wanted to know when I first started noticing a loss of memory. They asked what kinds of things I forget and other stuff."

I asked, "Did anyone comment?"

I just desperately wanted him to tell me the docs thought he was okay.

Other patients entered quietly, and I wondered what their illness was. It felt foreboding and depressing. It felt humiliating and daunting. I just did not feel like we belonged in an aging center. John and I were a healthy and active husband and wife who looked forward to old age sometime in the distant future.

It was a long day, eight hours in total, and I thought I had never been part of such a thorough and lengthy physician's exam.

This must be serious, I thought. *Or it could be serious*. I had no idea that this was the day that would mark the end of our lives as we knew it.

Finally, late in the afternoon, we were invited into a bright conference room. About five doctors sat around the conference table. A large screen hung in the front of the room and one doctor sat at the head of the table kitty-corner to John.

I sat next to him on his other side. We were both robotic. Part of me was sitting next to John. Another part of me was in another universe. I was impatient to hear the news, but at the same time I wanted to escape.

The doctors introduced themselves: a mix of specialties in aging and memory of which I have no memory, although the doctor at the head of the table was a neurologist and she ran the meeting.

She instructed, "If you look at the screen in front of you will see a picture of John's brain. It is from the brain scan you had completed previously. The doctor explained in a professional and non-emotional voice, "The gray parts are areas of atrophy in your hippocampus, John, which controls memory."

I thought, *It doesn't look like a lot of gray.* I also thought, *I never seem to understand what an x-ray or scan shows.* I just nodded and believed what I was told.

The doctor continued, "John's brain is losing the ability to remember things."

Then she described a summary of his tests, both written and verbal. She summarized, "John did well on his spatial tests, but he had trouble remembering words and being comfortable with his environment, like knowing what day and date it is."

She calmly reported, "John, you have mild cognitive impairment, which is consistent with early stages of Alzheimer's." It is hard to say either of us was surprised. We would not have even been in the room if we hadn't thought something was wrong. But we were both stunned.

John, in his jovial way, asked two questions: "Can I still drink alcohol?" "How long before I am a vegetable?"

She asked John, "How much alcohol do you drink?"

"I have a couple of glasses with dinner almost every night. Erica and I like wine. We kind of wind down each evening with a glass. It signals the start of the end of the day."

The doctor told John, "Alcohol is never good for you, but I am not going to tell you can't drink the wine you like so much with dinner."

I was then surprised at her straightforwardness with the *vegetable* question. She said, "On average people have between five to six years from diagnosis."

I asked, "What can we do to slow this down?"

She explained, "Exercise is the number one thing you can do for yourself. Good nutrition is also important. Walk every day. Get your heart moving. You want to get the blood flow to your brain. I will prescribe Aricept, which is supposed to slow down the progression of Alzheimer's. It is really the only drug on the market for Alzheimer's."

That was pretty much it. We left the building and silently and slowly walked back to our car.

I had a delayed reaction, because when the doctor said John had Alzheimer's it felt more like she said he had a cold. Only later in the day did I actually feel the pain-it stabbed my chest. I have no memory of our conversation on the way home.

Super Bowl Sunday

Sometime around 1979, I was walking down the hallway of Smith-Kline and a group of women were standing around giggling. My curiosity was piqued. I asked what was going on. Someone said, "Didn't you hear? Baccus is separated. He's single."

I had no idea that so many women were interested in John. "Why was I the last to find out," I thought, and "what does that mean for John and me?" I also thought this was not a giggling situation. A family's life was being turned upside down.

John and I had become fast friends. We went out for drinks after work, we lunched together in the park with colleagues or in a restaurant and we had our curbside talks about my relationship with Bob, or work gossip or just a little routine flirting.

One night it was just getting dark when I walked to my car to leave the bar. It was parked in a spot by itself. John walked with me. I opened the car door and slid into the driver's seat. I was smiling to myself. We had a nice time together. I rolled down my window to say, "Good bye."

John leaned into the window opening and gently kissed me on my lips. He said, "Good night. See you tomorrow."

A Promise Kept

Do I need to tell you how happy I felt?

I was not shocked when John asked me to spend a weekend with him as Super Bowl Sunday 1980 was approaching. The real question was two-fold. "Would I leave Bob for a weekend with John, and could I find someone to stay with Danny?"

I was in that space where I was annoyed with Bob all the time and knew ending our time together was long overdue, but we didn't fight and nothing forced either of us to face our truth. It was time for Bob to move out of my home. We were both unable to initiate the finish.

One day he told me, "Erica, I think I am going to write a book."

I responded, "Maybe you should read one first."

I had lost respect for him. I could not have loving feelings for a man I did not respect. The glow of the romance had worn off leaving us with the lights on our actual relationship—which was shallow.

So, I told Bob a lie. I told him that I needed some space (a 1970s word)—time away to think about our relationship. I asked him if he would take care of Danny while I was away. They could watch the football game together. It was going to be a good game—the Oakland Raiders vs the

Philadelphia Eagles. Bob agreed to be the good guy and I left to spend the weekend with John. I never gave a thought to my relationship with Bob because it was soundly over.

When I returned on Sunday night, I went into my bedroom to think about what to say to Bob.

He followed me into the bedroom and said, "I can tell from your face this is over for us." I nodded. He opened the closet door, pulled down his suitcase, packed his clothes and quietly left.

Courtship

We had an unusual courtship. I continued to see other men the entire two years John and I dated. John could never commit to me—he did not date anyone else—but he could not emotionally commit to a serious relationship, so I kept dating and I kept telling him about my dates.

I'd tell him things like, "I went out with Phil again last night. I had a decent time."
John questioned, "Where did you go? How often do you see him?"

"Oh, we just went to a movie and then dinner. I think I'm going to end it."

"Really? Why?"

"It's just not going to go anywhere. I'm not that into him."

I had been divorced since 1970 and he had only been separated for a year, so I understood he needed some time to understand his new life and new role as a separated dad. But I was in love with John. I knew that for sure so I accepted what I could not change. I knew I had to give him time, so while I could wish it were different, I was also not in a hurry.

I had spent the last ten years dating on and off, mostly men who were truly not marriage material. I was in no hurry to get married again. I was not looking for a husband or love. (I drove my mom crazy; she thought the only way I could be happy was if I "had a man.")

Those were the 1970s. I dated men who said out loud, "I'm not interested in a serious relationship. I am not looking to get married." I dated men who were not interested in kids. I dated men who wanted more kids and I couldn't have more. I dated guys who were just into dating to have a girl with them, but not to get to know her.

On and on it went. I took my breaks, but always returned to the scene. The truth is I wasn't ready for a serious relationship either. My divorce at twenty-five had taken the wind out of my sails. I had never been single so this was my time to figure out what I actually thought about everything.

I had a traumatic divorce and I needed time to regain trust. I needed to learn to trust a man again and trust that relationships could be good.

I had warring thoughts battling in my head. My mom was not so subtly pushing me to get married again even before I had a chance to mourn my marriage. I felt I needed time to recuperate and maybe have some fun. I knew in my gut the next time I needed to know the guy in an honest way.

But John and I grew together out of a wonderful friendship and amazing chemistry. We talked to each other. I learned about his life and he wanted to know about mine. I confided in him.

One night I was really scared to tell him my big secret. "I can't have any more children, John."

"That's okay. I have a son. You have a son. We don't need any more. I am interested in *you*."

John sensed my insecurities and treated me gently. When I worried about Danny, he'd tell me, "Erica, you are a good mom. Your instincts are good. Trust yourself."

When I felt down about not making enough money or wasn't in a high enough position, he'd reassure me with, "You are going to get promoted—have patience. You do a really good job. You are very smart."

He encouraged my need for independence: "Erica, look at how you moved to California. You came alone with a six-year-old kid, you knew no one, had no job, and now look at you. You have a great job and nice friends, and Danny is doing fine. Not many people would have the courage to do what you did."

He played games with me to get to know me better. One night as we were sitting on his bed, he said, "Close your eyes. Imagine you are walking down a path. Imagine a path you like. What is on the path? Then imagine you come to the end of the path. Who is there waiting for you? There is a house at the end of the path. What is in the house? Who is in the house with you? What does it all feel like to you? How would you like to change it?"

We took turns playing that game many times through our early courtship. It made me feel special and it made me feel like our relationship was special. The game taught us about each other. We learned to be gentle with each other.

It had been a very long time since I felt emotionally safe with a man.

John was the only man I ever knew who was happy for me when I succeeded in accomplishing something. When I got promoted, when I got a raise, when I sold an idea to a customer, John was the person who was happy for me.

He told me I could do it—whatever *it* was. And secondly, John was the only man who did not compete with me—to ensure he was better, stronger, smarter, funnier, whatever than me.

John was on my side. So, I could be on his side.

He was my best friend. He made me laugh. When John put his arms around me, I felt safe, loved, and happy. We could talk about anything and everything. We held the same social, financial, and family values.

John loved to argue. Sometimes I think he took the other side of a discussion just for fun. Sometimes the discussions helped me see the other side—see the world from a different perspective. Sometimes we held strongly to our own beliefs, but it was always interesting, because John was so smart and engaged with me in our talks. John was always present.

For example, John and I talked about Dan's future.

"I think college is a place where one can discover his/her interests. It is a place to become exposed to all kinds of ideas."

"Actually, Erica, it is a place to get a degree that leads to a job so you can make a living."

"Really," I said. "Then why did you take all those courses that had nothing to do with business?"

"Well, I never had a chance to just learn for the fun of it."

"So do you agree with me?"

"No, I do not agree. I still think the purpose of going to college is to ultimately get a job. I don't believe it is to become an educated person. You can do that on your own."

John and I had a lot in common. He loved kids and I had a son whose father lived 3000 miles away. We both thrived on the outdoors. I taught him how to snow ski and backpack. We rode bikes and hiked all over. We shared our appreciation for the outdoors. He understood how I felt connected when I smelled the pines in the forest. He felt it too. We shared that joy of being physical in or with the outdoors whether it was fording a stream, catching a fish, or making love with the stars and moon as our company.

He fished at campsites while I read books and ate his fish with glee. He always gave me the fish cheeks to eat-the sweetest part. That first summer I announced, "John, I am going camping. Do you want to go with me?"

"Sure," he said. "Where are you going?"

"I have no idea."

"Let's pick a place together."

I pulled out a map, closed my eyes and let my finger fall where it may. Yosemite! Cupid was on our side.

I had only gone backpacking once and that was with a friend who was an experienced backpacker. Given that I grew up in Chicago and never owned a sleeping bag, I decided to take a class at the local junior college in backpacking. Really! Most importantly, the class taught me what to bring on a backpacking trip. I made a list of everything we would need which gave us confidence to adventure into the wilderness together for the first time—both of us beginners.

John and I went to REI and stocked up on all the awful dry food we needed, all the cute little containers for food, decent air mattresses, and sleeping bags. We laid everything out on my bedroom floor, which was a very large room, and packed according to the list.

We used that same list over and over until finally we assumed we had it all figured out. Later on we even substituted real food for some of the dry food. I do wish I still had that list.

Yosemite became our place. We could go way up in the back country any time we wanted. It was easy to grab a wilderness permit spontaneously from a ranger in those days. We could go skinny dipping and make love on a rock and not worry about another person anywhere near. John once confessed to me as we were reminiscing that love-making on rocks hurt his knees. I could only smile and think how worth it—it was.

One night early on in our relationship, we were both reading in our tent. John had rigged up the flashlights, so they hung over our heads like bedroom lights. I was into my book when he said to me, "I could fall in love with you. You don't need me to entertain you. You are perfectly happy just reading next to me."

I guess for him that meant he could be free to be him. John's war cry was, "I have to be me." I learned to respect that need. I learned to give him the space he so needed.

As connected as we grew to be, John and I always had our own interests. He loved to garden and I loved photography. He built a train set in our garage and I learned to be a pretty good cook and a better baker. I enjoy time on my own. I *don't* need people to entertain me all the time. So, we worked as a couple. And, when it was that time of day to come together, we neither needed nor wanted other people.

We just wanted to be together. We were so good together. We only invited one person to ever backpack with us and that was our teenage niece, Anya, who belonged in nature. (She became a PHD biologist.) She came once (her first ever trip) and wrote her college essay about it. Other than that, backpacking was our thing. I can still picture us walking side by side on a trail having deep talks about the world, our families, our jobs. It was our time just to be.

What's On My Mind

October 1, 2020

It sits in the back of my mind like a constant concrete thought bubble. I don't even know it is there most of the time. Then I stop to think, "What is that nudging feeling on my mind?" and then I think, "Oh yes, that." I wish I could meditate it away. I carry John's illness with me like another leg or body part. I am getting used to it. Sometimes I force myself to really think about what is happening, but I can't seem to stay with it too long.

If I focus on it, I imagine so much sadness. I simply cannot lose my husband. And, yet I see that I am losing a little bit of him slowly but surely. Maybe I am too negative and he will never get worse than he is now. That would be a lovely thought.

I am learning what I believe is the true meaning of marriage. I am learning what it means to love in sickness and in health. I am learning patience, compassion, and kindness. If I try to put myself in John's shoes, I imagine horror. I could not have the resilience or the positive attitude he has. It is when I imagine this is happening to me instead of him that I get a real sense of the illness.

A Promise Kept

And most of all, I cannot believe it is true. It just can't be happening to us.

Mostly I feel like I just need to wait and see and meanwhile get and give extra hugs and extra I love yous, and extra cuddles.

Erica Baccus

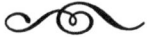

Gratitude

I look back on my life
And see love
It fills my heart
And makes me remember
So many hugs and I love yous
So many children for me to cherish
Thankful for my family
Thankful for my life
Thankful for my John

We Were Not a Match

John and I should never have had anything in common. My first husband, Don, and I were a perfect match—in theory. Same religion, same economic class, same educational background, same political views. However, we lacked the more important agreement on cultural values, personal and social values. Don's focus was on making money, being a financial success and proving to his dad he was a good businessman. I wanted to help people, especially kids, and build a close knit family.

John and I were the reverse. We came from completely different backgrounds.

John grew up in poverty. He was raised by a single mom on welfare along with three older siblings. He met his father once when he was thirty-eight. His hometown was in rural California. He was the only one in his family to complete a college education.

My parents, on the other hand, were upper-middle class, highly educated European immigrants who raised the four of us in Chicago to be a foundation for a close family. They hoped for us all to marry into similar backgrounds and raise a bunch of children. They wanted to replace the family that was lost in the Holocaust.

I did not see John's family home until after we were married. It was a good thing. I probably would have been too scared to marry him after seeing where he grew up. The house was an old army barrack turned into a structure that looked like a wolf could huff and puff and blow it down at any moment. Four kids slept in one room and mom had a bedroom. The kitchen where mom cooked liver and onions for breakfast had floors that sloped down towards the front door. It reeked of mold.

John's mom was mentally "off" but I could tell from the moment I met her that John was the recipient of her total love. Regardless, John was wary of his mom's behavior to the extent that he did not tell her we were getting married; he did not invite her to the wedding for he feared possible outlandish behavior.

John had tons of stories about his childhood that he told me and anyone who would listen.

"Hey kids, did I tell you the story where I almost died in the cave?"

"No Papa, tell us, tell us," they screamed as we drove in the car somewhere.

"Well, one day, me and Paul and Rosie decided to hike up to the cave on top of the mountain near our house. Paul was the oldest and Rosie just a year older than me. I don't know where Phil was that day. He usually came on all our adventures."

"Papa, how far up did you have to hike?" Owen, our oldest grandson, asked.

"Oh, it was a big mountain. But I was only about ten, so I probably thought it was higher than it was. Maybe a few thousand feet up."

"Whoa," the boys whistled.

"Well, we got up the mountain and there is a big ole leftover mining cave up there. So, what do you think we did?"

"I hope you didn't do anything scary," Noah, our second grandson, worried.

"Paul said we should crawl into the cave and look around. Paul was the leader cuz. He was the oldest, so we all followed him. First, Paul went, then Rosie and I went last. We had to go single file because it was too narrow for two people at once."

"Was it dark?" Noah wanted to know.

"Haha, yes it was dark because we didn't have our flashlights with us. We couldn't see our hands in front of our eyes. It was perfect for a game of tag. Of course, it was Paul who suggested we play tag, but I thought that was a very cool idea.

"The three of us crouched low and ran-crawled to catch the one closest to us. It was pretty weird in there. Wet with spider-webs and a very low ceiling. Rosie screamed every now and then and Paul and I laughed at her."

Owen pushed on. "So, you had a fun time?"

"Ya, it was fun until I was running away from Paul and couldn't see where I was going. I was one move away from stepping into a crevasse and plunging down to the bottom of the cave. I didn't even know there were breaks in the cave floor."

"Oh my god," the boys breathed out together. "What happened then?"

"Just as I was about to fall into the darkness, Paul grabbed my shirt and pulled me to him."

"Was your mom going to be mad at you?" Owen wanted to know.

"Oh, we would never tell her about it. We never told her anything we did on our adventures. They were our secrets."

He loved his chaotic, wild childhood. He and his older two brothers and sister ran around the hills and caverns all summer long without any intrusion from Mom. They slept outside most of the time and came home for food when they were hungry. They stole watermelons from neighbors' yards, collected cans to sell for a nickel at the store and hosed themselves off in neighbors' sprinklers. They were feral.

I spent eighth grade through high school in a fancy suburb of Chicago where my friends belonged to country clubs, went to camps each summer and most kids had their own cars to drive to high school. College was not a question of whether I would go, but where?

John and I both believed family was a priority. We had strong work ethics and neither of us cared about "having more." We had what we could afford and that was fine. We were happy whether we had financial setbacks or financial successes. We both believed in helping other people, telling the truth, and giving each other freedom to stretch our minds and imaginations. We kept learning, changing and accepting each other's newness. Sometimes, it took work and time to catch up to the other one, but we believed in each other. These are the things that made us work.

Our different backgrounds spiced up our lives making us more interesting to each other- match or not a match.

Day To Day

This thing is with us every day now. It feels alive. It grows and changes and inserts itself into our lives-unwanted but ever present. Sometimes John and I each ignore it in our own way, but it is there.

John's brain is changing. It makes us sad. He speaks of losing himself—losing the person he was. I see it too. He is not the same John, but I am also not the same Erica. I have been more able to focus my life on my priorities and more open to laughing out loud with John. I have learned to become a real sports fan—especially worshiping the Warriors, which has made John so happy.

John gave me permission to fail, to take risks and embark on new adventures. I could never have started my own business if John hadn't told me I should go for it, because he thought I'd be good at it. I would never have moved to Boston with John if he hadn't given me the security blanket where he promised we could return to California any time I wanted. I would never have forged a river with twenty-five pounds on my back if John hadn't reached his hand out to teach me, I had nothing to fear. I have changed for the better, but my brain is not diseased.

I never expected John to change in this way. I never expected him to become less independent, less engaged in life, less able to read books or follow the plot of a TV show. I do not think of John as "less" but the reality is he cannot maintain new information in his head. I have outsourced my brain to John. I do his thinking for him. I plan his golf date every week with his buddies. I make sure he has the clothes he needs for whatever events are on the calendar. I narrate a basketball game when I realize he is not tracking. I remind him about current news, the stock market, and our financial status.

I didn't think about those things before because I took our life for granted. Well, not exactly for granted, because I used to tell John we should count our blessings. Our kids were doing well and didn't need help from us. Our grandkids were adorable, smart, funny, and loveable. And John and I were healthy, happy and financially secure. We loved where we lived and enjoyed all that the beautiful Bay Area offers.

What more could we ask for?

Since John's diagnosis, I have become a mistress to the task. I think and plan to make sure I have not missed doing something important. Does he need a neurologist appointment? Has he eaten today? What time is his golf date? I think for John because he cannot. I remind him of our social events several times a day. I remind him to go to his exercise class. I am in a constant alert mode to ensure I see new changes in his behavior and attitude.

And then there is fear. I suppose it is fear of the unknown or perhaps it is fear of the known-what we have read and heard about. I believe I am learning to live with fear. It is a quiet little spot somewhere in my brain that says, "The shoe is going to drop, Erica. Watch out!"

John and I don't know what will happen tomorrow, but in this case we know that as this thing progresses, it will not be good. We know his brain will deteriorate and he's going to become less and less functional. What we don't know is how fast or when or what it will look like.

So we stay in the present.

We remember that each day is a gift. We remember to hug each other and to say, 'I love you.' We find the goodness of our lives in each other—in our friends and the people we love so dearly.

It is hard to stay positive and not focus on the future—on our limited time. The future is not a place where either of us wants to hang out. It is scary and sad. We help each other. We remind each other that *today* is our day, that today is what we have and no one knows the future. I try to remember the teachings of Buddhism. I am merely a novice meditator, but the lessons are good: "Stay in the present. Suffering comes from wanting things to be different from what they are." I can relate to this conceptually, but executing the right behavior is difficult.

John is better at being grateful for what we have had. I, on the other hand, want more. I want more of our life together. I want more love from John. I want more fun and affection. I want more normal conversations with John. I want more laughs with him and I want to make more memories with him. I want more. I am a lousy Buddhist.

With Alzheimer's, one loses one's personality, ability to function, dignity, love of life. And still, we don't really know exactly what will happen tomorrow. Maybe John will get hit by that proverbial bus—and sometimes I wish for that. I mean, I don't really want that to happen, but sometimes it all gets to be too much. Sometimes, I know John would just like it to be over. Once he was standing in our bedroom with his head in his hands leaning against his dresser with his back to me and he said, "Just shoot me, Erica. Just shoot me now."

I felt so helpless. I thought, *This is now getting to the point where his suffering is interfering with his life. I want to take him in my arms and make the pain go away. He has taken all the hits on his body and brain with little complaint. He deserves better.*

I thought I had paid my dues in my early life. I had lost two pregnancies, two brothers, a marriage and both parents. I thought I was going to get out of this later life with ease. We are both healthy and active. We ski. We play golf. We hike. We ride bikes. I thought it would just keep going like this until our turns came to a stop when we were really old.

I was wrong. It has nothing to do with dues paid. This is simply what life is. And now I am learning to accept this thing. It is here to stay. In our home, in our bedroom, in our conversations, but it is not in our love. We have love all to ourselves.

John and I have always had an intimate relationship. We are social people with lots of friends, but our first choice is always to be with each other. I don't know if that is unusual, but we both love cuddling and spooning each night. It was my safe place. John is my safe place. Our love is like an armor that protects us from the outside world. All we have to do is hold hands, watch TV, or smile at each other and nothing can intrude on our peace and love.

"Why are you so far away from me," John asked as we relaxed in bed.

I moved closer to him. "I love looking at you. You are beautiful. How come you never changed in all these years?"

"Ha ha, John. Beauty is in the eye of the beholder. But thank you. Let me turn over and you can cuddle me."

He put his arms around me and held tight. "Not so tight, John. I feel like I'm in prison. Just loosen up a bit."

He relaxed his arms. "Ah, that feels wonderful. Now I can sleep safe and sound."

As the night passed and he turned the other way, I followed him. Back and forth we went in our sleep. Spooning all night.

In a video I took a few days before John died, I asked him, "John, what were some of the things we did in our marriage you liked best?"

Without thinking for a moment, he answered, "Sleeping with you, Erica. I have always loved cuddling with you." He must have read my mind.

A Promise Kept

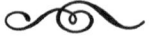

The Audacity of Hope

Hope dares to edge in
Brave and bold
Without regard to danger
Forgetting to announce herself
How dare she?
Hope knows no boundaries
For what are we without her?
Necessary to our hearts
Needed by our brains
She doesn't give up
Doesn't give in
Wraps us in her loving arms
To see beyond the tears
To live beyond the fears.
We feel the soft silence of the peace she brings us.

The Splits

Our dating life drifted up and down. In the beginning, John invited me to his great big empty house where we smoked dope, cooked fried baloney sandwiches, ate peanut butter sandwiches and made exhaustive love until I needed to go home. John's house was completely empty with the exception of his bed. (He gave all the furniture to his ex-wife.)

He grew marijuana plants in a closet with very clever hanging lights from one end of the closet space to the other. I was pretty impressed with his creativity and ingenuity and his marijuana. We spent most evenings on a blanket on the floor in front of the fireplace. It never once occurred to me to ask why he didn't buy a table or a chair. We had memorable times in that great big empty house.

Each time I rang his doorbell he greeted me by grabbing my arm to pull me into his embrace. Always greeting me with a big smile and his hearty laugh. I knew he cared about me.

But after a while, just as I was getting very comfortable with our relationship and I'd start to wonder where it was headed, John ended it. I remember three specific times.

Time 1:

I had spent the weekend at an Esalen retreat in Big Sur. (Another 70s thing.) I left Big Sur feeling confident and powerful. *I am woman. Hear me roar.* John was meeting me at my house. We spent the evening talking in front of my fireplace just about what my experience was like and what he had been doing while I was gone. I had thought about what I wanted to say to him all the way home from Big Sur. I knew it was risky, but I felt it was important that he knew my truth, and I felt so empowered by the weekend retreat that I took the risk.

I said to him, "I am going to tell you something and you do not have to respond. I just need to tell you how I feel. I took a deep breath and squeezed out, "I love you."

Then I watched him stand up and silently leave my house. It was weeks before we spoke again.

Time 2:

It was a Sunday morning in Spring 1980 and we had just made love. I was feeling so happy and cared about. I was leaving for Germany soon after that to travel with Danny, whose soccer team was scheduled to play there. Because John and I were keeping our relationship a secret at work, I asked him, "John, how are we going to handle our relationship from now on at work?" What will we tell people?"

It seemed to me that we had had a change in the seriousness of our relationship. He responded by saying, "It's not a problem since I'm not going to see you anymore when you come back from Germany."

This, of course, did not last long after I returned home, but it hurt, and it was another red flag that John was not moving in the same direction as I was.

The thing about John's breakups is that they were never caused by an argument or discontent with each other. I was never angry with John for breaking up—I was sad. I was disappointed and I missed him terribly, but I was never angry.

Time 3:

I found this next chapter of John's life to be somewhat off-kilter. John was a college-educated bio-tech manufacturing manager, and at the time he quit his job he was a marketing manager. He quit for reasons I either never really understood or don't remember. There was a lot of disgruntlement, anger, hurt feelings and resentment on John's part. I have no idea what upper management thought.

At the time John quit working for SmithKline I was actually his assistant product manager. John had grown bored with being the packaging manager in the manufacturing department when an opening occurred in marketing. He called me one night.

He said, "Hi, Erica. Guess what. I have been offered a job in marketing as a product manager. Linda offered it to me. I don't know what to do. What do you think? You know I'll be your boss. Do you think we can work together like that?"

I was all over it. I said, "Well, are you sure you want to leave manufacturing?"

He responded, "Yes, I've been doing that for so long and my degree is actually in marketing. I'd like to give it a try."

I wanted to work for him—that meant I could be with him all day and it would be so much fun. I also thought the change would be good for him.

I said, "I'd love to have you as my boss. I think we can make it work. We just have to behave ourselves."

John took the job and I became the person who helped him get everything done on time. "On time" was not something John ever regarded as highly important, while I was raised by a father who thought on-time was thirty minutes early. We were a good team. He knew how to be a product manager and I knew how to write reports, which he hated doing. He knew how to charm customers and vendors and I made sure projects stayed on schedule.

It was so much fun while it lasted.

One day, Linda, the director of product management (a woman whom I considered a friend) called me into her office and told me quite directly that she knew John and I were dating and if anything went wrong with the arrangement at work, it would be me who would get fired. I was the woman. I was the assistant. I was surprised but not worried. "Okay, that is fine with me. We are not going to do anything wrong," I assured her.

We continued our working lives together, ate our lunches together, had after work drinks together and spent weekends together. I was very happy. I thought he was too.

Then, squabbles broke out between middle management and upper management. I was not part of either, but John was. He was very vocal. He became very unhappy and short-tempered with the status quo and up and quit one afternoon. Boom!

He was gone. No warning, no discussion. I recall feeling very sad for John.

I took over his old job at my present salary. Gotta love how that works. I did his job and got paid the assistant's salary. That would not fly today. John fell into a depression and spent most of his time alone at home in his big old empty house. I loaned him money so he could have time to figure out his next move and I tried to encourage him to look for a new job.

Well, he found a new job, but not one I would have expected. Instead of going back into biotech management, he decided it would be a good idea to sell camper shells all over the West Coast. He drove from dealership to dealership, small and large, north to south on the coast and inland in California. He ran away. This time it seemed to be forever.

Selling camper shells required him to travel so he took this opportunity to explain, "Erica, I am going to be traveling all over the West Coast. It's going to be difficult to see you anymore."

This was a serious ending and I believed it was real. He left me. I had just lost my best friend and the man I trusted with my person and my love.

Below is the letter John wrote to me in October 1981. It is filled with love and I received it knowing he did not want to hurt me. However, my sorrow filled a cavern. I truly believed I would never see John again.

As I read this letter now, more than forty years later, I am struck by how he says goodbye to me. He could have written this just last year on July 26, 2023 before he died. He has taken me with him.

A Promise Kept

Dear Erica,

I remember you reading your diary about how you were going to survive last summer when Danny left for Florida. You started out, "Today is the first day…" Today was my first day of truly being alone and I survived actually rather well. I am pleased that you didn't call because it makes what we both have to do a little easier.

I suppose you're wondering why I would sit down and write this letter (you know how I love to write!). Well, here is the reason. I had to do what I did last night. I didn't like doing it, but I had to have my release to start my life again. The part I didn't like was to minimize what we had together and I want you to know that what we had together will always be a part of me and it is a lovely, wonderful part. Thank you for being you. It really helps to know that you have the same feelings. I guess "growing up" never is easy and the people in our lives often get hurt in helping the process, but I want you to know that it was worth it. I am going to go farther and I know that you will too.

I'll never be far from you in spirit and if you ever need to use it, just as I will, sit back and think that we both could really be ourselves and that there is someone in this world that thinks that was pretty neat.

Perhaps this is the first goodbye in my life that is truly an honest one because I am not leaving you. I am simply taking you with me. I wish you the best.

Love, John

Nothing Is Forever

When I was twenty-four, I lost two pregnancies within eight months of each other, which ultimately resulted in my not being able to have any more children. I had wanted five—one more than my mom had. I was raised to be a mother and now I had only one, so I had to readjust my vision of who I was besides the fact that losing a child for me, even one in utero, was devastating.

My mom had counseled me when I was in high school.

"Be a teacher, Erica. You like kids. If you are a teacher, then you will have the same vacations as your children. You'll be home in time to cook dinner for your husband."

Or, "Erica, be a teacher. You like kids. That way you'll have a back-up in case your husband dies. You'll have something to fall back on to support yourself and your children."

I heard this mantra repeatedly. It burned into my brain. I'd go to college, get married and have children. I'd have a teaching degree so I could have a career AND raise children. There just was never any question that I'd have children and be a good mother. I vowed to have four or five kids, because I had three siblings.

My mom also urged me on because she and Dad lost so much family in the Holocaust. "Erica, we are a small family. Daddy and I had four children because we wanted to make up for our losses in the war."

I believed I needed to continue the regeneration of our family. So, when I was told I could no longer have children, I became depressed. I hated feeling like I was depriving my son of siblings. I hated the idea that my home would not be noisy and busy with kids' stuff. I hated feeling sorry for myself among friends who were repeatedly pregnant.

If I am not the mother of a big family, then who am I?

The summer of 1972 answered the call of my soul. I found what it meant to feel alive again, traveling through Europe with a friend. I found that Mother Nature fed me and I found what I needed to be happy. But I had no idea how to turn my discovery into action.

Sometime in the late winter of 1973, my older brother, Jim, called me.

"Hi Erica. I need to tell you some news."

"Hi, Jim. I hope it is good news."

"Well, it is for Sigi (his wife) and me, but I don't know how you will feel."

"Now you have me really curious. Go ahead."

"You know my residency is coming to an end and Sigi and I are looking for places to live. I am looking for a permanent position to practice pediatrics."

"Ya. I know. I am happy for you. Your career is getting ready to take off."

"Yes, but the thing is we are looking at places in California. We are going to move to California. We want to get out of Chicago. I have a list of cities I am going to interview in."

I paused and without thinking anything through, I said, "Jim, I'm going with you."

This was the angel on my shoulder moving me towards what I instinctively knew would be my home. It would be my home that would offer me what I found climbing the mountains of Switzerland, wading in rivers in Austria and breathing in the sunshine and sweet smell of the forests all around Europe.

My cat kept him company as he pulled the U-Haul. I took his dog as my companion on my month-long cross-country trip to San Jose. Jim was three years older than me and my protector. We were always best friends.

Thus began my and Danny's new life. It is now fifty years later and I am forever grateful to Jim for taking me with him, for helping me start over in a strange and weird place, and for being my protector.

Jim and Sigi had two gorgeous kids. Anya was a year old and Ted three when they relocated to San Jose. Jim was a pediatric cardiologist who was beginning his career there and so excited about starting his life in the sunshine.

One morning nine months after our move, Sigi called me sounding urgent. "Erica, Jim is sick. Can you come take care of the kids while I take him to the hospital?"

No questions asked, I said, "Of course, I'll be right there."

I grabbed Danny, ran to the car and drove the eight miles to Jim and Sigi's house. I found Jim unconscious on an ambulance gurney and Sigi barely holding herself together. She left with the ambulance. I still had no idea what was wrong, but both of my brothers had been sick all their lives, on and off, due to a genetic disease.

Neighbors who came over when they saw the ambulance told me, "Erica, go to the hospital. We will watch all three kids."

I arrived at Santa Clara County Hospital and was met by a physician in the emergency room. He said, "I'm sorry to tell you this. Your brother Jim has died."

I punched the doctor while I sobbed. He asked, "Would you like to see him?"

"Yes." He took me around the corner where my brother lay seemingly asleep. I crawled into bed with him and hugged him goodbye. He was thirty-three years old.

My younger brother, Terry, lived with the same disease. He survived several cases of pneumonia and many life-threatening bouts of flu. This blood disease compromises one's immune system so the body cannot fight off bacteria.

Terry was almost sixty-one when the phone call came. John and I needed to fly to Utah to say goodbye—Terry was in the last stages of lymphoma. He and I had just talked the day before and he sounded great. His decline was shocking.

He was still alive and conscious when we reached the hospital. Terry reached his hand out to me, "Thank you for coming, Erica."

I held his hand, choked back my tears and said, "Terry, I love you. Of course, I would come."

His three children, wife, our sister and brother-in-law and John held vigil for a few days knowing this was the end.

Throughout it all, the one focal point that kept me from dropping too far into grief or too long was my child. I needed to care for him, so I had to put my despair in a place where I could visit rather than live.

So yes, when John left, I was both startled and empty and now needed to adjust my life again. I needed to accept that he was not in my life. I mostly remember standing on the sidewalk in front of my house the morning he said goodbye, feeling sad and so alone. I stood on my sidewalk in front of my small house waving goodbye and wondering how I would get through this.

Near the end of 1981, I was at my desk at SmithKline. It was in the marketing area, a large room that was front and center. The senior managers all had offices along the perimeter and I had a desk facing a wall in the center area with my back to my new boss's office. We had no computers and we used dial phones. My desk had a screen around two-thirds of it and me.

One afternoon my phone rang. When I answered it, I heard John's voice. I had not heard from him since he had left a few months earlier. I was excited, happy and nervous. I tried with all I had in me to stay calm and I was over-the-top curious about why he was calling.

"Where are you? How are you? What's going on?"

He said, (and some things one never forgets) "I am calling you from the Golden Gate Bridge. I am wondering if you would meet me for a drink after work at our place?"

I said, "Yes! Yes, I'll meet you for a drink." I felt tingles in my body, but I was also very curious about why he wanted to see me.

I was so happy to see him. He looked so handsome and happy to see me. We sat at a table in our very familiar bar and John ordered us two glasses of white wine. We sat next to each other shoulder to shoulder rather than across from each other. I had to turn my head to look at him. Or maybe we sat across from each other and I looked away from him. I just remember I had to turn my head to look him straight in the eye when he started talking to me.

This is what he said.

"Erica, I have been driving all over the West Coast and every place I go I think of you. I remember all the beautiful trips we took together and I see you everywhere. I realize none of this means anything without you in my life. Will you marry me?"

I had to catch my breath and replay what he asked. He sat quietly waiting for my answer.

With my face turned slightly away, I finally responded, "John, you have never even said you liked me. And now you are asking me to marry you?" Then I paused. "I can't do that."

There was still no mention of his love for me. I suppose one could interpret what he said as saying, "I love you," but I wanted to hear him say the words. I wanted clarity.

"Will you at least think about it?"

I looked straight at his eager face and beautiful blue eyes, "Yes, I'll think about it."

From that point on I could think of nothing else. I was dating another man and I couldn't care less what happened to him or to our relationship. I kept trying to figure out what was the best thing to do for my life and my son's life. There was no doubt in my mind that I was in love with John, but I did not trust his feelings for me. I had been single for a long time now—eleven years—and I knew one thing for sure: I was not going to have another bad marriage.

John kept pestering me for an answer. He called and called to ask if I had decided. In the meantime, the other man I was dating started to become jealous of John and he wanted me to stop talking to John. I finally got so fed up with John and the "other guy" and told them both to go away and leave me alone.

One night I called John and said, "I am so sorry, but I have decided I can't marry you. I just don't trust that it will work."

I broke up with the other guy. That felt good and it felt right for me. I felt relieved even if I didn't feel happy about saying no to John. At least I made a decision.

One Saturday not long after the proposal, I was lying on my living room floor listening to Neil Diamond—our favorite—singing, "Hello Again," our song. I was totally immersed in the music and feeling very nostalgic and romantic. It was a sunny day. I had my glass front door open so I could see through the door from where I was laying. All of a sudden, I heard a car racing by the front of my house. It was John. He tossed a scrapbook onto my front lawn, yelling, "This is what you are throwing away. Look at what you are throwing away."

I ran outside and picked up the scrapbook. It was the one I made for him as a gift. It was filled with photos from our first Yosemite backpacking trip together. It was filled with love and joy. I carried it into my house, sat down and looked at the pictures thinking, *this whole thing is so sad.*

John left me alone for a few days and then late one night he called me to ask, "Will you meet me at Denny's just for a few minutes? I just need to talk to you."

It was late and Dan was sound asleep in his room. He was thirteen, so I felt I could leave him alone for a short time. I drove to Denny's, which was less than five minutes from our house, and met John in a circular booth. We ordered coffee.

He begged, "Please, Erica. Marry me." It was late and I needed to get back home to Danny and my bed. Again, I sadly said, "John, I am so sorry, but I can't. It just won't work."

The pressure was overwhelming, and I felt really bad for John. Was I throwing the best thing ever away? Was I losing my one chance for a happy marriage? How could I know?

John tried one more time to convince me to say yes to him. By this time, I was getting pretty good at saying no. He had asked me to marry him three times and I said no three times. After the last time, he got very frustrated and said, "That's it, Erica. I won't ask again. Goodbye."

Time passed with no more phone calls from John. Then on the evening of November 30, 1981, my sister called me. Danny and I had just trudged into the kitchen from a ski trip in Tahoe. We were taking our ski jackets off when the phone rang. I answered and Judy, who is fifteen years younger than me, screamed while crying, "Mom's dead." She abruptly hung up the phone, leaving me holding a dead receiver in my hand trying to process what she said.

My mom had early-onset Alzheimer's. She was 63 when she died. No one really knows when she first started showing symptoms. In those days, no one really heard of Alzheimer's. My father, an outstanding anesthesiologist and first-rate medical doctor who also happened to be an excellent diagnostician (sorry for all the superlatives, but they are real), had to research medical books to discover what was wrong with my mom. She had been starting to have memory glitches and exhibited confusion.

One night I was somewhere with my parents, and we drove to their house in the same car. My mom opened the trunk of the car to retrieve her dry-cleaned clothes and I saw a stack of medical books in the trunk. My mom pointed to the books and said, "Daddy has been looking to see what is wrong with me. He says I have a disease that is going to make me really stupid."

My heart broke. I was most upset about how she described the disease—*making her stupid*. My mom was a really smart person, but she grew up in old-fashioned Europe, where it only mattered if the son was smart. Her brother, my favorite uncle, Walter, was also a doctor. She grew up in his shadow feeling totally unimportant and everyone just assumed she "wasn't that smart." Or actually, it was like no one cared if she was or wasn't.

But I knew she was a very capable woman who was actually an excellent writer. She took English classes at a college in downtown Chicago. I was in high school at the time and a good English student. She wouldn't turn a paper in to her instructor without asking me to proof it. She was mostly concerned about her English grammar and punctuation. I can still remember reassuring my mom telling her that her paper was really good. She asked me if I was sure, because she did not want to be embarrassed. She brought her graded papers to me and they were always A and maybe a B thrown in every once in a while.

She undertook this challenge for herself—for her own self-esteem. I don't know that it helped, but I saw first-hand that my mom could easily compete with American college students. So, when she declared that she had a disease that was going to make her *really stupid*, I knew how that must have hurt her. This was her button. This was what she had been fighting all her life. I so hope my dad didn't actually use that language—that it was her interpretation.

I was living in my house in San Jose, CA with Danny. One day in October, I was talking to my mom on the phone. She lived in the suburbs of Chicago. I realized during the conversation that she could no longer remember Danny's birthday. Danny was her first-born grandchild, and she adored him. I thought, "Wow, if she can't remember Danny's birthday, she must be further along in the disease than I knew."

It was hard to gauge what was really going on two thousand miles away from someone. We had no Zoom or FaceTime and long-distance phone calls were expensive. I decided that I needed to visit. Her birthday was October 5, so I bought myself a ticket and flew to visit her.

I was stunned. She could not write a check to pay for groceries, because she had no idea what date it was. She couldn't find anything in her kitchen and the contents of her cabinets were a complete mystery to her.

My mom was a superb knitter. She knitted beautiful coats, dresses and sweaters and now she had no idea what to do with the needles she would need to hold. As a chain smoker, she needed to put her cigarettes out in an ashtray. She had several cigarettes going at once—each on fire in its own ashtray in rooms throughout the house. But she knew me and could hold a normal conversation. I spent a lovely long weekend visiting with my mom and she was so happy to be with me. We did not often get time alone, so this was precious for both of us.

"Erica, how is Danny doing? I miss him."

"He's fine, Mom. He is in eighth grade. He's playing a lot of soccer and is getting pretty good. I hope he'll make the high school team.'

"Mom, why aren't you knitting?"

"I can't, honey. I can't remember how to do it."

"I am so sorry, Mom. I love you."

The last thing I said to her that weekend was, "Mom, I met a man I really like." My mom was desperate for me to be with a man—she wanted me to get married. She thought it was the only way I could possibly be happy. It didn't matter that by this time I had been single for eleven years. I gave her a gift by telling her I met someone I liked.

But my mother did not die of Alzheimer's. I last spoke to her on Thursday, November 26, 1981. I called to say happy Thanksgiving to both my parents. My mom didn't sound well. I asked how she was, and she told me that she had been sick and was just now starting to recover. She died on November 30. She had a virus in the lining of her heart. Just five days after I spoke with her, she died suddenly while driving her car. My mom's caretaker was in the passenger seat. She reported that my mother said, "Ow!" and slumped over the wheel. She died instantly, and the caretaker had to grab the wheel and pull over to stop the car.

After Judy called, I ran to my bedroom, threw myself on the bed and sobbed vehemently and loudly. My lovely, smart but scared son said, "Mom, call John."

Those were the most important words anyone ever said to me, I think.

I had John's phone number for his new house. He had just rented a room in a house in San Jose which he shared with several others. I had, of course, not seen it but I knew where John lived. He wanted to stay in touch with me so he called me once to let me know where he was moving. I called him crying on the phone, barely able to get the words out. He asked me in a very concerned but gentle voice, "Erica, what's wrong?"

All I could squeeze out between sobs was, "My mom died."

He just said, "I'll be there as fast as I can."

John arrived at my house while I was still shedding tears on my bed. Danny left me alone—poor kid—he had never seen me like this, so I am guessing he had no idea what to do with me. John came into my bedroom, gave me a hug, and went into action. He asked, "What do you need?"

I said, "I don't know. I need to pack and figure out how to get to Chicago."

He started by doing my laundry, packing a suitcase for Dan and me, bought airplane tickets for us and called Sigi to ask if she needed him to get her plane tickets too. He said he'd stay in our house until we returned home. I accepted everything he offered with gratitude.

Dan and I flew to Chicago on December 1. We stayed for the funeral and several days after to mourn with family. John stayed at my house the entire time.

I thought a lot about him during my stay at my parents' house and on the flight home. I thought about how short life is, how fragile, but mostly, I thought about how John was there for me when I needed him most. Very few people in my life had been there for me when I needed them most and certainly not a man of romantic interest. I thought about how scared I had been to commit to another serious relationship forever. I thought that maybe—just maybe—this was the time to start trusting. That meant trusting in my own judgment and trusting my love for John and trusting John's commitment to me and Danny.

I was greeted at our door by John who was holding a clay pot with a plant in it and a piece of 8½ X 11 paper folded in half with these words in John's beautiful, expertly printed handwriting:

"...Far beneath the

bitter snow

Lies the seed that with

the sun's love,

Becomes the rose."

"I can't think of a more appropriate time when the lyrics of "The Rose" have had such meaning. Please accept this gift as a means of remembering that love survives when all else has gone. –John."

The plant held a white rose, which John planted in my backyard. It bloomed for the first time in April just in time for me to carry it as my wedding bouquet on April 17, 1982.

John gave me a dozen white roses every year on April 17th for 41 years.

The night I returned from Chicago, I asked John, "Will you ask me that question you had been asking me?"

He took me by my hand and walked me into the living room and asked. "Erica, I love you. Will you marry me?"

This time I said, "Yes."

I felt a little nervous, but mostly truly happy and ready to do this thing I had been avoiding for a very long time. It scares me now to think how close I came to losing my life with John.

For the next few days, I kept asking John, "Can I tell our friends and people at work that we are getting married? Can I say we are engaged?"

He answered so confidently, "Yes, tell anyone you want."

I really did not accept that this was a real thing—that we were actually going to get married. Each time I asked him, he told me to go ahead and tell anyone and everyone I wanted.

The real challenge was telling my dad and the rest of my family. I had kept John pretty much a secret from my family. I had not wanted to tell them about break-ups or get anyone's hopes raised that I finally *found a man*.

So, when I called my dad I said, "I want to tell you that I am getting married."

In his Hungarian accented gravelly voice, he demanded to know, "And may I ask to whom?"

Danny was happy, relieved and excited. He had been waiting for John and me to come together for quite some time. He used to ask me, "Mom, when are you and John going to get married? Are you going to get married?"

John and I actually started to make plans for a wedding. We decided that since my dad would be coming to California in April for Passover, we should combine it with our wedding so he would not have to make two trips to the West Coast. I got out the calendar, found the dates for Passover and planned our wedding date to be April 17—right after the holiday. That simply is now my second or tied for first happiest day of my year—right up there with the day Danny was born.

Wedding Bells Rang

April 17, 1982. Our do-it-yourself Chuppah stood in the middle of our living room. John sewed the covering on his old Singer sewing machine and then built the stand. It was one of the first miracles I saw him accomplish. I came from a family where changing a light bulb was a feat. No one could do anything mechanical or had any handyman talents. John was a genius with all of it. In forty-one years, I never stopped being impressed with what John could build and fix. When our grandsons were young and they wanted to build something, John could take them into the garage and help them turn their dreams into a reality.

I chose the material for the Chuppah, a silky blue thick material with white trim. The colors coordinated well with our living-room furniture and blue is the color of the Israeli flag. I am not a religious person and I don't belong to a temple. I am one of those culturally Jewish people who just *feels* Jewish. I grew up in a Jewish home surrounded by Jewish friends and my parents escaped the Holocaust. Being Jewish is part of my identity. My parents were not religious either, but I was raised in a home where conversations about Hitler and concentration camps happened routinely. I wanted to be married by a rabbi and John did not care. He was raised as a Catholic by a very religious mother, but John was a *fallen* Catholic.

In 1982, it was really difficult to find a rabbi who would perform the marriage ceremony for an interfaith marriage. After searching for quite some time, I did find a rabbi who agreed to marry us. He was blind in one eye and had only one arm, but he had the credentials to conduct the service and that was all that mattered.

Home from the pre-wedding dinner at Sigi's house, I changed into my white knee-length, long- sleeved white dress. Danny sat on the edge of my bed watching me while I was putting on finishing touches to my make-up. He was pretty thrilled as he watched me get dressed. I asked him, "Is Don ready?" (Don was his father's name.)

He looked at me smiling and said, "Mom, you must be really nervous."

I have always loved my relationship with my son. And at that moment, I just wanted to hug him like crazy. He knew me. He understood some of what I felt—probably better than anyone else.

When the time came for the actual wedding to happen, sometime in the early evening when the sun was still shining, Rabbi Robin arrived late to our home. He was just late enough to make me anxious, but not so late that it mattered to anyone. There were seventeen people sitting and standing in our living room crowded around the chuppah. Mostly, family and a few very close friends were invited to share in our incredible joy. My sister stood in the back of the room next to the bookshelf that held our stereo system. She was responsible for playing the records at the right time. She was only twenty-three. I don't think she took her job too seriously, because I remember she forgot to turn on the music that we had chosen for after the wedding vows were spoken.

John and I chose "Hello Again" as our wedding march song. Our plan was to walk from our bedroom to the living room in step with the music. As many times as John and I practiced it—mostly for fun—I could never figure out which beat of the music we were supposed to start on. I stood next to John, asking, "Now?"

I was wrong every time we did it—and on that very special evening, I was wrong.

We took our first step when John smiled and looked at me, holding one of my hands while I held my white rose in the other hand and he said, "Now, Erica." We marched the short walk and were only interrupted once by the toilet flushing in the middle of our song. My friend Jean did not know we had started, so she chose that moment to use the bathroom. It didn't matter. I'm probably the only person who noticed it.

We arrived at the chuppah. Danny stood on my left and Kyle stood on John's right. Rabbi Robin stood in front of the four of us. I promised John, "I give you my love, I give you my friendship and I give you all of me."

Even though we had not told each other what our vows were going to say, John's were almost exactly the same as mine. Throughout the first nine years of our marriage that we lived in that house, I took John to that spot in the living room when we argued about how to be fair to both of our sons or when he continued to spend his days fishing off the pier instead of finding a job. I did it to remind him of our vows and to remind us both that we promised to be each other's friend—to be married to each other with love in our hearts and to allow each other to be—just to be.

We lived by those words for 41 years. We held nothing back and sometimes it got to be a little much. Sometimes our emotions get away from us. We had to take time to go to our own spaces, to take a breath and let our feelings breathe.

But we learned what each other's buttons were and learned to respect each other by not pushing them. We learned how to disagree with each other and not say things we would regret forever after. We learned to not let hurt feelings get swept under the carpet—so we talked to each other. We learned that making sure the other person was happy was the best and easiest way to ensure that each of us was happy. We gave ourselves to each other, we gave our love and our friendship to each other.

We stood in the chuppah as husband and wife with smiles that could light the room. Someone handed us a glass of champagne and I told Judy to play the song we had chosen for this moment, Bette Midler's "The Rose."

John always thought we had the best wedding ever. He thought it was the most beautiful, meaningful and lovely one he ever witnessed. It was small and sweet. It was personal. Our sons stood next to us, each on one side, under the chuppah that John built. My white rose from the garden was lovely and fragrant, and we played the music we chose over and over in the days and years that followed. We held hands each time one of those songs came on.

I wrote my thoughts to John each year in an anniversary card and he did the same. More than once I repeated my vows to John on a card.

Erica Baccus

My dear John,

I promised to give you my love, my friendship and all of me. It has been my joy to share me with you. I look forward to a lifetime of love, friendship and the amazing fun we have together.

With Love,

Erica

Family Man

John happily adopted my family. He kept up his phone relationships with his brother and sister and a visit here and there, but it was my extended family he chose to be his. My sister became his, my nieces and nephews became his, my brother became his.

Of course, Kyle and Lori and Drew and Haley became a part of our whole family right along with John. Everyone welcomed John into their lives and hearts. He was the fun person, the person one could confide in and the one each could love with no strings attached. Because he gave what he received.

He carved the scariest pumpkins with the kids, provided the best belly-full-of-jelly laughs and built the tastiest gingerbread houses at Christmas. He willingly played poker with the older ones knowing he would lose. He played fantasy baseball with my brother and went on spring training trips with him each year. He hugged everyone like a big cuddly bear and listened carefully when someone felt like confessing a problem.

Thanksgiving has always been my favorite holiday. I have been hosting Turkey Day for almost fifty years insisting on doing almost all the cooking myself. I roasted a turkey in the oven and John barbecued one in the backyard.

A Promise Kept

John's favorite activity on Thanksgiving was to round up everyone to play tag football on the street in front of our house. We live in a quiet neighborhood where very few cars pass by on a holiday. The little kids and big ones formed teams with John leading the charge. I watched from the window when I could sneak away from the kitchen. It was a 1950s kind of fun.

A few years ago, John's turkey was on the barbecue. Our nieces and nephews were keeping him company outside while he tended the turkey. Apparently, John decided he could leave it and start the football game.

"Come on, everyone. Let's go play football out front. Dan, go get the Nerf ball."

"I'll get Ted," Anya yelled. "And my mom and Aunt Louise."

John threw the ball to Noah and screamed, "Catch it, Noah. Run."

"Yay, Noah."

Everyone cheered.

"Who is going to run for the extra point?" Dan asked.

Finally, John said, "Time out. I need to check on the turkey." Just a bit later, he came running into the kitchen, grabbed a bottle of red wine and yelled at me, "The turkey's on fire."

"Oh, no, I gasped. Oh, well," I thought. I went down to the backyard to survey the situation and found John bent over a black turkey scraping away some of the charred skin. He confidently told me, "Don't worry, Erica. It will be alright."

Dinner time. John carved my roasted turkey and then turned to his creation. He sliced a piece off for me and I tasted it. "John, that is the best turkey I have ever had. What did you do to it?"

"Simple, Sweets. I just cleaned it up a bit and poured a bottle of red wine all over the bird."

For some reason, this memory sticks out in my mind. It is so perfectly John. Ready to play, organizing the fun with the family with no worries about the small stuff. It will all be okay.

He knew he could fix the problem.

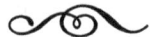

Sounds of Silence

I was married
To a very loud man
Who laughed and grumbled and chattered away
He tinkered with tools to saw and to sand
His voice and his giggle and his love came to stay
Our home neither quiet nor dull
But crammed with ideas exchanged and what happened today
How I miss the sound of life that can happen
When love gets time to play.

Ski Story

Our first married winter, 1982-83, was a snowy one. One of the attractions that drew me to California in 1973 was that I could ski here. My six-year-old son and I could escape to the mountains together, buckle up those godawful boots and cruise down a powdery mountain 8000 feet above sea level.

John, my California-native new husband, had never locked skis onto his feet, but like most everything else, he was gung-ho to try. We had rented a ski cabin for the winter on the east shore of Lake Tahoe in Homewood. Our first outing was a weekend when I asked John, "How much did it snow last night?'

He laughed and suggested, "Look out the window. Look out the bathroom window. You can't see out cuz the snow dumped itself all the way up to the top."

"Okay, let's put on our warmest clothes and get going."

"All I have is jeans and my long underwear. That will be fine. It's actually getting sunny outside now. It's going to be a gorgeous day."

At the top of the mountain, I asked, "Are you ready? We will take it slow. First and most important, I'm going to teach you to stop."

"Okay, I'm game."

"John, get behind me and watch me. Then you try, but wait for me to stop and I'll tell you when to go."

I started out in the pizza formation everyone uses to learn to ski. I slowly skied down a bit and then turned my body uphill to stop.

"Erica, where is your weight when you turn?"

"I'm not sure. I have to take a turn and think about it. I just do it by feel. But I think it's the downhill skiing."

"Which one is the downhill ski? Is it the one downhill when you start or when you finish the turn?"

"Well, your weight starts on the downhill ski and transfers to the uphill. Just ski behind me. Do what I do."

He tried to watch me and ski. He managed to not fall and got a bit better each try. But then John asked again, "Where is your weight when you go into the second turn?"

"I have no idea, John."

I started to laugh. I am the one who John taught to measure distances by deciding how many trees there are to the object or how long something is by imagining how many six-foot men it is.

Here I was, Miss Watch Me and Do It trying to teach Mr. Physical World how to ski. We fell down on the snow together, threw fluffy white balls at each other, and laughed at our differences.

Boston

May 1991. John and I were packing for our first trip to Europe together. We were headed to France for three weeks. My career had taken off once Danny graduated high school, and now I was a marketing manager for a high-tech publishing company. I was not thrilled with this job, but the pay was really good.

My phone rang as I was closing my suitcase. The voice said, "Erica, this is Riley. How are you doing?"

Riley was a former colleague of mine who worked for the rival high tech publishing company. I liked Riley but certainly could not imagine why he was calling me.

"You are leaving for Europe tomorrow?" he asked. I could tell this threw him for a loop and he was thinking things through really fast. He said, "Erica, I have something I need to talk to you about. I want to make you a really great offer."

I was skeptical, but curious. Riley never did anything that wasn't good for Riley and I knew he liked to do things over the top.

"Erica, I want you to come back to IDG. I want you to be VP of Marketing for Corporate. But you have to live in Boston."

"Riley, we are getting ready to fly to Europe tomorrow. It's our first vacation in a long time. I cannot even think about this now."

"How are you getting to Europe?" Riley asked.

"We fly to New York and then on to Zurich."

"Great, I can meet you in New York and we can talk about this."

"Riley, we are leaving for vacation for three weeks. Can't this wait? Besides, I don't want to live in Boston."

"Erica, I'll meet you on the shuttle bus from domestic to the international terminal. We can talk there."

"Riley, this is nuts."

"Just hear me out and then you can go on your trip."

We arrived in New York and just as we were ready to step on the bus to the International Terminal, an Irish ball of energy in a blue suit jumped on the rumbling crowded bus. Riley stood on the bus hanging on to the strap above his head. All smiles, like this was a normal thing to do, he shook hands with John and said, "Hey, man. Good to see you."

Then he looked at me and pitched me with a heavy hand. "Take the job, Erica," he offered, "and become the VP of marketing for a world-wide publishing behemoth. Your salary will be something you never dreamed of, and IDG will pay for your relocation and pay your rent while you look for somewhere to live with John."

I thought, *Take a breath, Riley.*

"But you have to decide soon, because we need to fill this position fast. We are building a new marketing/sales force and we need you to head it up."

"Riley," I moaned. "I can't make a decision now. I am getting on a plane for our first trip together to Europe. At least wait until I return. You are asking a lot from John and me."

"Okay, we will talk soon." And with that, the bus came to a stop, and he jumped off and disappeared.

John and I looked at each other. We had no idea what to say or do. This was a fantastic career move, only in the wrong place. We decided we'd put it all aside and enjoy our trip to France.

Ha! Easier said than done, especially when Riley or the VP of IDG kept calling me every other day to see if I had made a decision. So, I had to think about my options constantly while trying to relax. John was pretty much, "Whatever you want to do, Erica, we will figure it out." I finally demanded that IDG leave me alone until I get home from our trip so we could enjoy ourselves.

Once back in San Jose, I told John I had made my decision. "I am going to turn them down. I moved to California because I wanted to live in California. I don't want to go back to those dark gray winters. I know what the snow and the cold is like. You don't. This is my home."

"Okay," John said, "but think about this. What would you say if you were ten years younger? Would you go for the adventure or say, 'No?' I've never lived anywhere but California except Vietnam. I think it would be fun to have a new experience. We will have a good time together." He easily convinced me to give it a try. I hoped to see the fun in this new venture, but I felt more agitated than pleased. I choked back tears anticipating leaving my beloved California and vowing to be more positive.

"Agh," I thought, "I don't know. This is my chosen home. I'll go under two conditions. 1) We don't sell our house, so we have a home to return to anytime we want. We can rent it out while we are gone. 2) At any time for any reason either one of us can raise our hand to say I want to move back to California and the other person has to agree with no recriminations." I was so scared of our decision. Rather than feeling excited about an opportunity, I felt dread.

John agreed to my terms. I called Riley to tell him that, yes, I accepted his offer and thanked him. He was delighted and instantly told me what date to plan on arriving. He also promised to get me a hotel room until I found a place to stay.

Riley gave me a date to arrive in Boston. He was now my boss so it was no longer my choice. Reality hit. John and I had a good-bye party for our friends. We invited everyone to visit us wherever it was that we were going to live. I sat with John on our front steps reminiscing about our lives in San Jose. He said, "It has been a sweet life here. We will build a new one together in Boston."

It was summer so I packed up my cool clothes, bought an airplane ticket, and hesitantly said good-bye to my home for the past eighteen years.

It was hard. John took me to the airport where we kissed and hugged good-bye, but Riley provided airplane tickets for John to come to Boston on weekends. We needed to look for a permanent home together. So, I knew we would not be separated for long.

John stayed behind to rent out our house and pack it up for the cross–country relocation. John became the traveling spouse.

I found an apartment on Commonwealth Avenue in Back Bay, walking distance to my new office in the high-rise on Boylston and Exeter. My window looked out on the Public Library, the very first in America. It was June. It was hot. Two hundred fifty thousand college students had just emptied out of Boston. The city was filled with U-Hauls and college kids excited about being done for the year.

I was enamored at first. My new temporary home was an old brownstone with an English garden in front. No air conditioning and dark hallways and small narrow spaces were the trend in all of these brownstones which made quaint streets in Back Bay. I had never lived anywhere alone, and this seemed like fun for a while. I even thought it was cool to go to the laundromat. I was really trying hard to adjust and have a positive attitude. I decided if I was going to do this move, I should give it a 100% try. Even though we had a "safe get out" agreement, I knew I needed to think of this as a new adventure and think positively.

I loved Boston's history. It is our history—America's history. I walked to Paul Revere's house, the Boston Common, the cemetery with tons of famous people buried there like Ben Franklin's parents, Sam Adams, John Hancock, the victims of the Boston Massacre, and many more. The famous Trinity Church was also across the street from my office, which was also on the route of the Freedom Trail. There was much more to the city and its historic past, but Boston is also home to the iconic Fenway Park and Newbury Street, the elegant shopping district, also walking distance from my new apartment. My location was superb.

However, Boston summers are also noted for their humid, hot, mind-numbing days. On weekends, I walked to the mall in Copley Plaza to watch movies—any movie—in an air-conditioned theater. On weekdays, I worked from early morning in my comfortable air-conditioned office until it got dark. I picked up a pastrami sandwich at the nearby deli and went home to call John after the sunset.

Kathy was my work friend and became my best friend. She lived in a gorgeous home on several acres outside of Boston and she adopted both John and me. She helped us find a house to buy, introduced us to all her friends and showed us all over the city. She made life in Boston livable.

But the New England culture was very foreign. Kathy could trace her roots back to the Mayflower, which is cool, but why is that important I often wondered? Riley, my now-new boss, took me out to meet clients. As we were driving one day, he described each client we were about to meet and included from where each had graduated college.

I said to him, "Riley, do you know you keep telling me where everyone graduated college from."

"Ya," he said. "Of course. It is important to know."

I countered, "Riley, I can't tell you where any of my best friends went to college, no less work colleagues."

"Hhmm," he replied. "That is definitely weird."

The elevator in our office building opened right into our lobby. A receptionist sat at a desk directly facing the elevator so she is the first one you see when you exit the elevator. One morning shortly after I arrived from California, I was wearing a skirt and blouse with a necklace of colorful wooden beads. "Morning, Erica," the receptionist said.

I answered back, "Good morning."

She said, "Lose the beads."

"What?" I asked in a shocked tone.

She explained, "This is not California."

This same receptionist asked me how my house hunting was going. "What neighborhoods are you looking in?"

I said, "Jamaica Plain and Brookline."

She said, "You can't live there."

She was pretty adamant but I thought she must know something I didn't since I was new and she was a native. I asked, "Why not?"

She explained offhandedly, "That's where all the Jews live." I never bothered to clue her in to my own heritage, but I was wary of her and other comments from then on. I felt like I needed to watch my back.

I grew up in the 1950s on the south side of Chicago and went to an elementary school where I was one of three Jewish kids in the school. Our neighborhood was all white with two other Jewish families on two very long city blocks. I was used to antisemitism. It scared me and offended me. I was always afraid to answer back because I did not want to embarrass the person who was persecuting me. I am still trying to grow out of this ridiculous sense of "being nice" even when I know I am not the one in the wrong.

It wasn't just bias against Jews. I was invited to the opening day at Fenway Park that spring. The sales guy for an ad magazine took me as his client. I sat in a really good seat, thrilled at the idea that I was at Fenway. I looked around the stadium and something felt very strange. It took me a few minutes to figure it out. I said to my host, "The stadium is all white. Everyone's the same color here?"

Totally unimpressed with my question, he answered, "Of course, baseball is a white man's game."

These insults to my value system made an impact. They festered in my mind while I tried to think this is just a different culture from California. I tried to tell myself to forget this and adjust.

Finally, in late August, we had closed on our new house in Wayland, eighteen miles northwest of Boston. John moved out of San Jose and we began our new life. He managed to get a good manufacturing job really fast with a biotech company, so things were falling in place.

New friends of ours invited us to brunch in New Hampshire one Sunday morning. John and I were in awe that you could brunch in a different state. In California, you can drive for hours without leaving the state. People thought I was weird for living so far from my work—it was eighteen miles. At home, I drove on three major freeways for at least forty-five minutes to get to and from work. Things were different. I knew there was an ocean in Boston, but darn, it was hard to see it. The beaches were private so houses blocked the ocean views. Not so at home. Public access to the ocean beaches in California is a must. Trees were so numerous in Boston it was hard to see the horizon at any time except winter when the leaves had fallen to the cold brown ground.

We lived on the leaf-peeping trail which meant during the fall all kinds of tourists drove past our street on Rich Valley Road. We lived in the neighborhood of the Ws: Wellesley, Westin, and Wayland. I understood why hordes of cars drove through Route 20. The scenery looked like a romantic comedy setting with sunshine and brilliant reds, yellows, and oranges everywhere.

We lived a twenty-minute ride from Thoreau's Walden Pond, a few blocks from the first one room schoolhouse and about six miles from Concord which is the location of the "shot heard round the world" and the beginning of the American War for Independence.

Our first winter arrived. All our neighbors gawked at John when he so excitedly got out his brand-new blower to brush away an inch of snow. Our back-yard boasted three tall, statuesque evergreen trees all in a row which we could see from our kitchen window. We called them the dancing ladies; they looked like a chorus line. It was a Christmas card setting when the white snow dusted the green statues. Our home was cozy and warm and the biggest I had lived in since I was divorced in 1970. When the first blizzard hit and the power went out, the neighbors called to say, "Bring over your food from the freezer. We'll have a potluck." We became close friends with these neighbors who invited us in to share their hospitality, introduce us to other neighbors and show us their Boston ways.

Time passed and my job became routine. Riley, who was so excited to hire me, started hassling me about small things. I missed my old friends. I began to feel like if you don't know my son, who was away at college, you can't know me. How can we be friends? The holidays were tough for me while I was so far from any family. The winter was long and dark. Four o'clock rolled around each day and the light disappeared. The long gray winter started to wear me down. After I arrived in California, people asked me, "Why did you leave Chicago?" My answer was always the same: "February." I hated the brownness of Chicago's winter.

On occasion, I had to fly back to San Francisco for business. Each time the plane began its descent, I looked out the windows to see a wide-open horizon with mountains reaching up to a sunny sky. I felt my whole soul reach up to touch the beauty and openness of the San Francisco sky. I smiled inside each time I landed.

Slowly, I slowed down. I became lethargic and sad for no reason. I lost my desire to work or see friends. I crawled into my bed and thought about nothing. I did not even realize there was something wrong with me.

Finally, when I could no longer get myself out of bed to dress for work, John started to worry. He pulled me from our bed and pushed me into the shower.

"What are we going to do, Erica? You can't go on like this."

I called it. I cashed in on our agreement.

"I can't do this anymore, John. I need to go back to California."

I lasted only eighteen months. For so many reasons, the Bay Area became my home that I could not leave. I am just one of those people whose environment affects one deeply. I need the mountains and the ocean. I need the sunshine of California. I need it all for my mental health.

Boston turned out to be great for my career and we made some very good friends. John loved living in a new environment complete with all four seasons. Like most other things in life, nothing is all good or all bad. I'm glad we went but even happier we returned to California.

I returned home in February 1993. Elated, exuberant, high on life, I called my best friend, Jean to let her know I was back. I had found a great job at a high-tech ad agency in San Francisco and a wonderful place to live. John stayed in Boston to sell the house and pack us up again.

He never complained. I am not sure he understood my need for the environment we had left behind, but he saw me suffer. He always had my back. I flew back to help John with last minute moving details and on a blizzardy windy cold April day, we said goodbye to New England.

Lox and Bagels

I liked making lox and bagel sandwiches for John. I liked doing it because he got so excited when I told him, "I bought lox for dinner tonight." It's such a simple thing, yet it brought him joy and became a routine for us.

I often planned to have these sandwiches for dinner on Warriors game nights. We tried to watch all eighty-two season games together on TV. We ate a lot of lox and bagels. I had to buy the smoked salmon at the deli on Chestnut Street, and the cream cheese and red onions at Safeway where I get my staples, but the tomatoes needed to be perfect, so I made a special trip to a market with really good produce.

One night in 2022, we had lox and bagel sandwiches for dinner while we watched a Warriors game. The game was almost over when John said to me, "I'm hungry. When are we going to have dinner?"

"John, we already ate lox and bagel sandwiches, but if you are hungry, you can have more."

He said, "Okay," and turned around to walk back to the kitchen to make another sandwich. He returned with a handful of Oreo cookies and a glass of wine.

A word about tomatoes. Most tomatoes in a grocery store taste like cardboard and are often too soft and grainy or they are too tough and hard to bite into. Tomatoes are one of my favorite foods, so I am really picky about them. My favorites, of course, are John's from his greenhouse when they are in season.

I have learned through meditation to focus on the food I am preparing. It feels good to take my time and feel the process. I try to pay attention to cutting, stirring, and chopping and think about how it feels and smells. It is quite rewarding to find peace in my work in the kitchen.

Toasting the bagels was pretty simple, but John liked his bagels to be golden brown. I opened the cream cheese and spread it carefully across both halves of the bagels. I made sure the cream cheese covered the bagel evenly—no spaces left untouched. The lox came next. I did not skimp on the lox, after all, it's the main reason for the sandwich and I wanted the taste to seep through all the other ingredients.

I took my knife and slipped it under each slice of salmon to get one piece at a time. I laid it carefully on top of the rich white cream cheese and continued one slice at a time until the salmon was piled relatively high—folded neatly across the bagel.

Days of Our Lives

It got harder as the days and months and years passed. We could both watch the disease progress. Sometimes we didn't acknowledge it. But by the time a year or eighteen months had passed, we were becoming more direct and honest. I'd say things like, "John, think about today. Today is a gift. We have each other today." Then he'd hug me.

Or John would ask, "How much time do you think we have left? Erica, you are going to have to tell me when you think it is time."

Almost to the end people didn't really notice the depth and extent of his memory loss and accompanying symptoms. But I remained on high alert all day—every day. It was as if I was taking inventory of his brain capacity each hour—each day. Sometimes I thought, "He's not so bad. He can hold a very articulate conversation with me." Other times I thought, "He is declining too fast."

He stopped having opinions. His judgment couldn't be trusted. He would say he wanted X one minute and Y the next. He'd say, "We must watch what we spend. I want to make sure you have money when I am gone." Then five minutes later, "Erica, where is our next vacation going to be?"

I had to learn to decide what he wanted for him, because he didn't remember or he just could not decide what he wanted. I can't tell you the number of times he'd change his shirt before going out. "John, why did you change your shirt?" I'd ask. "You looked nice in the one you were wearing." John answered, "I didn't like it. I don't like the way the collar looks."

During the course of John's illness, there were times when I became very frustrated. Sometimes I fantasized about running away, and sometimes I wanted to hide from the world. I didn't want to run away from John. I just wanted to run away. I hesitated to spend time with friends, because my brain was just overfull with Alzheimer's Disease. It was always at the forefront of my mind, but I didn't want to talk about it with my friends. What could they do?

I thought, *I can't do this anymore. But, Erica, it could be so much worse. I can't talk to people—nothing but Alzheimer's will come out of my mouth. A beach in the sun would be nice now—me and the beach and a good book. But I don't want to go without John. I always want John with me. I need to stop wanting what I can't have. There is no escaping our reality.*

Because John's judgment was questionable, I needed to be responsible for decision-making. Important things in our life became my responsibility. Doing the taxes, renting out an empty apartment in our building, getting a repairman for a tenant's needs, and managing our investment portfolio all became my responsibility alone and it seemed like it happened overnight. The weird part of all this was that John did not question this. He wanted to know what I was deciding, but anything I did seemed to be okay with him. Strangely, this was not comforting. I needed his knowledge—his advice—his opinion. I got nothing.

He still took meticulous care of our garden. John knelt on the sofa every morning to look out the window of our sunroom to check on his garden. I used to ask him, "Are you watching the grass grow?"

He'd bring me up to speed. "The plum tree needs pruning" or "I need to fix the sprinkler system" or "It's time to plant the tomatoes."

Then he'd get off his knees, put on a sweatshirt and go down our back stairs into his garden. That would be the last I'd see of him until I realized he forgot to come in for lunch. Then I'd make him a sandwich and surprise him with it.

Sometimes, on a nice sunny day, I'd join him in the yard. With a book in my hand, I'd wander downstairs to visit John. "Maybe he'll sit with me for a while," I thought.

After he rested for a bit talking with me all the while, he'd jump up and say, "Gotta get those limbs down." Or, "I need to put a scarecrow up cuz the birds are eating all my cherries."

It gave me joy to see him work in the yard and build a beautiful sanctuary for the both of us.

Sometimes John had trouble regulating his emotions and I told myself not to take any anger from him personally—that it was the disease talking. And it was because ten minutes later he had no memory of being angry. Once when we watched TV, I changed channels without telling him I was changing. He yelled, "Why did you do that? I get to have a choice, too." He was right. "I'm sorry, John. I just wanted to check something out. I put it right back to where we were." I tried hard not to make John feel less—less of a man, less important, less capable—just less.

A Promise Kept

I bought a package of dry-erase boards. Each morning I erased the board from the day before, wrote today's date on the board and a list of events for the day:

1. It's garbage day

2. Exercise with Max at 2 p.m.

3. Warriors game at 5 p.m.

4. Dinner with Cheryl and Tom at 7.

Then I signed each message with a heart and *I love you* and some silly happy face.

Sometimes John wrote messages back to me. "Have a nice day, Erica. I love you." I liked that. He was having fun with our message board. The board worked well. It took some time, but John got used to going into the kitchen to look at the board when he wanted to know what was happening that day. Often, he checked in on it several times a day.

Then, of course, there were days when the board was useless. He couldn't remember what he read five minutes before, or he couldn't remember to look at the board. John could not remember that he could not remember.

It was in the summer of 2021 when I realized that I would never have my happy life again. It all happened so fast—I thought we had so much more time. When I thought about how John felt, I was terrified for him. I loved him so much and I did not want him to go through this pain.

In September 2021 John and I took a five-week trip to Spain and Italy. It was probably a bit too long for both of us, but as I look back, I remember how we both grew to appreciate Spain. We spent four weeks driving through that beautiful country. In spite of the difficulties due to John's illness we had a memorable and enjoyable vacation. It was all worth it.

I kept a bit of a journal on the trip. I wrote then that John was getting worse. I drove one thousand miles in Spain and he could not help with directions, he could not use my iPhone to help navigate, he could not remember yesterday and sometimes not even an hour prior. He knew he was getting worse and that was the worst part. I always imagined his pain when I thought about how he must feel. John had always been so adamant about being his own person and now he was recognizing his own decline.

Journal Notes:

9/25/21: We drove into a 15th-century medieval cobblestone village. Streets barely big enough for a car and tourists filling the street. I couldn't find the hotel and it started to rain. I stopped the car in front of a garage that I thought was the hotel. I asked John to get out to see if he could find the parking lot. Meanwhile a man was yelling, "Mi casa" at me. I rolled down my window and he repeated, "Mi casa." I apologized for blocking his house and then he spoke to me in English. He told me the hotel was two doors down. I pulled into the parking lot and realized John had disappeared.

I left the car to look for John in the street and he was just standing where I left him. I called him and he walked over to me. But he didn't know what happened to me. He had been sitting inside another man's car thinking it was ours.

I wished I could have been a better person for him. I wished I could have been more patient. I wished I could have given him more comfort and taken away his pain. John had always been such a truly good person. He never once uttered anything like "Why me?" or "How can this be happening to me?" Not once throughout his illness did he articulate any self-pity.

He needed a lot of downtime and I again felt like I was losing him. He was disappearing much too quickly and much faster than I expected. Sadly, he stopped having conversations with me. Yes, we could talk about what we were doing in the moment or I could describe to him what was coming up, but he couldn't start a conversation with me. I wrote in my journal: *I miss my husband. His personality is dwindling away little by little and watching it happen hurts so much. I am sad for John—I am sad for me.*

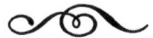

John

Laughing, loving, lively was he
Lonely am I
Losing himself into all he'd do
Loving him took my heart and brain
Last one to stop playing - he went on
Long ago I learned this is him
Let him go I think
Let me go he willed
Lovingly we embraced.

Doing It Myself

I had reached 50 and I was growing frustrated working for men who claimed my ideas as theirs, in places where integrity seemed like last on the list of priorities, places where quality of work could not survive against politics and places that counted beans instead of brains. John encouraged me to change the game.

"Erica, start your own business. You can do it."

"But John, I don't know how to manage a business. I've never done anything close to that."

"Erica, you are smart and experienced. You can do it."

I decided I could give it a try. I had been working as head of market research for a large high-tech ad agency in San Francisco. As part of my job, I hired and managed focus group moderators who conducted research for our agency clients.

One night after the first focus group was finished, but before the second one started, my moderator told me, "I am so sorry, Erica. I am not feeling well. I have to go home."

I took a minute to digest this news and said, "Of course, go home. I'll do the next group."

Carolyn was surprised, "You are going to do the group?" How are you going to do the group? You've never done one before."

"Well, I don't have a choice."

I walked into the focus group room knowing full well the clients were seated behind the mirrors. They would be watching me. Hopefully, I wouldn't mess up too badly. I'd hate to tell my boss that we needed to refund their money.

I took my seat at the head of the oval table and informed everyone, "Good evening. I'm Erica Baccus and I'm going to be your moderator tonight. We are here for you to help me understand the strategy you use for creating security in your IT. Everything you say is confidential. I am very interested in hearing what each of you thinks so I look forward to hearing from all of you. Let's start with you introducing yourselves to the group and to me."

All of a sudden, I felt totally at ease. I thought, *It is just like trying to get eighth-grade students to discuss a story we had read when I was teaching- to elicit their thoughts and why they held those thoughts. I can do this and it's fun.*

I asked questions such as, "How do you secure your network and describe a recent breach of security?"

"Can you tell me about the project that prompted you to buy security upgrades?"

Respondents answered and I even got a cross-discussion going.

A variety of responses helped me understand the depth and breadth of the marketing problem my client was facing.

Best of all, when I went into the back room to see if the clients had more questions, they did not. Instead, I heard, "Good job, Erica."

The group was successful and I had launched myself into a new career. I took a year before I made the leap, however. I spent that year figuring out cost structures, exploring how to obtain clients, and practicing moderating. When I felt I was ready, I resigned from my safe, secure job and went home.

It was 1996. We had been back from Boston for three years now. John had started a small business of his own. He was selling manufacturing machines as a rep for a few companies, but also, he was building and selling his own machines.

His favorite client, Henry, was the owner of Yank Sing, a renowned dim sum restaurant in San Francisco. Henry's company made its own sauces in his building in an iffy part of the city. He happened to have some open office space which he offered to John for an extraordinarily low rent. Henry told John, "Look, you can put your machines in the window and there's plenty of space for your manufacturing. You need to get out of your house and have a place for business."

John happily accepted his offer and created a professional space for himself and his machines. Once a week, Henry made sauce in his gigantic kitchen right behind John's spot. The scent of garlic took over the entire building on those sauce-making days, but otherwise it was a perfect location.

Homeless people sat on the curb in front of John's window. Of course,

John befriended the regulars, who protected his car parked in the driveway and ensured dangerous-looking people didn't bother John. Cigarette butts and empty liquor bottles had to be cleaned up each morning. Sometimes marijuana smoke eased its way into the open windows, but none of this bothered John. He was comfortable and happy on Howard Street.

John told me one day as I was typing away on a TV table in our sunroom, "Erica, Henry says you can have the loft space for an office if you want it. He'll let you have it for almost nothing,"

I looked up at him and said, "Let me think about it."

John took me to the building to check it out. I climbed the staircase and as it turned a corner, there it was. Instant love. I could see beyond the peeling paint and scratched floors. I saw my new creative space—my place for my business. It was a very large open space that my eyes followed to four beautiful arched windows. A second much smaller room with a sink and cupboards and bathroom was perfect for a kitchen area. All I would need is a refrigerator, coffee machine, table and chairs.

John saw me light up and said, "I can paint the walls, fix the floors and polish them, and put in new lighting."

I asked, "Can we put shelves all around the room?"

"Yes, of course."

I had a vision. I did not want anything with a corporate feeling. John and I went searching for the right furniture—the kind that fit my idea—on Market Street visiting all the antique shops. He understood exactly what I was looking for with something appropriate for working but something cozy and homey. We bought antique tables and desks that I chose for my two future new employees and myself and area rugs for each table or desk. These served as the boundary for each workspace. No walls or cubicles or Staples office furniture.

John worked magic and created a beautiful new space for me. He knew exactly what he and I both wanted and knew how to do it. I worked hard and long hours almost seven days a week, especially my first year. On Saturdays or Sundays when no one else was working and all was quiet, I drove to my office, clicked on my lights and looked around.

"This is all mine," I thought with pride.

And there I sat next to my windows typing away at my new computer for several hours all in the effort to get Baccus Research started.

John worked downstairs and I upstairs. We often drove to work together in the morning, stopping to get doughnuts and coffee at our favorite French cafe. John handled the money side of my business for me, so that was one less thing I had to do. My business demanded I travel. For much of the time, I was somewhere else in the world for about half of the month. John took over all the household tasks that had to happen: grocery shopping, laundry, taking care of our cat, paying bills and on and on. All so I could do what I wanted to do without guilt, and so we had time for each other when I was home.

Baccus Research was successful from the start, even though it took me years to relax and not think we were failing every month. I could never have done it without John's encouragement and support.

Fifteen years later I retired. I had the best boss ever.

Vietnam

John was drafted into the Army in Vietnam in 1966—the beginning of Vietnam. He lucked out and was not in the infantry, but Vietnam was dangerous everywhere. The stories we heard were gruesome.

John did not talk about Vietnam unless someone asked him. Then, he could go on for hours about his stories:

"One night I was in the bunker with another guy. It was our job to guard the camp. I was crouched in the foxhole and I saw something. I saw it move. Maybe he was one hundred yards away. I aimed my gun at it and waited. While I waited, I took another hit of my joint."

"Were you so scared?" I asked.

"Uh, not so scared—mostly just a lot of adrenaline going on and I needed it to stay alert."

"So, go on."

"My buddy and I stayed up all night long waiting for the enemy to do something. Guns pointed, we both watched as he just sat behind a bush and didn't move."

"Couldn't you ask someone else to come help?"

"No, the rest of the camp was asleep and we couldn't make any noise. Finally, dawn started to break and I could see the outline of the body better. I started to think I wasn't sure the guy was a Viet Cong. Then as the sunlight brightened a bit, I put my gun down, turned to my foxhole mate and said, 'It's a goddamn rabbit.'"

John told me they were mortared every night.

"Ya, it became routine. We had no idea when it would hit or who would get hit. We lived with the idea of dying every day."

One of John's jobs was to fly supply missions to Saigon in a helicopter.

"Ya, I liked flying in the helicopter. I volunteered for the job."

"But that was really dangerous, right?"

"Yes, helicopters got shot down all the time. But for me, it was a way to get off base and be somewhere different. I hated having to be in one small area for so long. And Saigon was cool. I got to spend a night there each time I went. I used to sit at the open door of the copter and hang my feet over the edge. We'd fly over killing fields and I saw death everywhere.

I learned to NOT be afraid to die."

John's Journey

John took a different path from me. He was happy with his own business for several years and then grew tired of the stress.

"I don't know how much longer I can do this, Erica. It's the same stuff over and over again. I tell my customers what they need, and they don't listen. Then they need a new machine or they say fix it, John, and I need it tomorrow. There has to be a better way."

I kept telling him, "You need to set boundaries. You just can't please everyone all the time. You have to learn to say no."

"I gotta go all the way to Redding tomorrow to deliver a machine. I just hope it works when I get there. I'm going to stop in Napa on my way home to talk to the jam-manufacturing guys. They want to talk about filling honey now. I'll be back late tomorrow night."

Then, "Erica, I think I want to turn off the lights."

"But John, you've worked so hard to make this work. You want to just walk away from it?"

"I know, but sometimes it is just time for a change. What do you think?"

"Well, you've been doing this for years now. I kinda think you should take some time to let it sit before you do anything."

"Well, I have a lot of hours in the car. I'll see how it feels in my gut."

He took some time off and eventually decided to return to working for the corporate side. Only this time, he chose a cosmetics start-up company close to home. He was responsible for all the manufacturing. I liked his job; John was having fun and he brought home cool samples of the soaps and creams he was helping to manufacture.

As time passed, management changed in the small start-up. The company started to become bureaucratic, and the fun began to fade. Each day he came home with another story of a political mess and fewer stories about manufacturing.

I should not have been surprised. One evening when I came home from work, John greeted me with, "I quit my job."

"What? "You did what?"

"I quit my job."

"But, why? And you quit without talking to me about it?"

"You knew I didn't like it."

"Yes, but who likes their job, John?" I argued. "You're supposed to find another job before you quit. You don't just quit."

"Well, I did."

"Now what?"

"Well, since Gretchen has to be on bed rest for the next two months, I'm going to take care of her and then when the baby is born, I'll help with the baby."

Gretchen, our daughter-in-law, lived with Danny in the building we owned in our garden apartment which was below us. She, not only was my son's wife and the mother-to-be of our first grandchild, Gretchen also worked for me. So, I was her mother-in-law, her landlord and her boss. One might think this was a prescription for failure—somewhere along the line, but Gretchen was and has always been easy to be with. Her no-nonsense upfront directness worked well with mine. Somehow, we managed to make it all work with love and humor.

John knew my buttons. He knew that I would not object to his plan if he replaced it with taking care of our kids and soon-to-be grandchild. I thought, "That's okay. They can use the help and now it will be easier for him to take care of our home when I am away for my business."

Gretchen was pregnant with her first child when John quit his job. She had preterm labor that caused the doctor to tell her she needed to take a leave of absence from work and stay off her feet.

John also knew that it would be easy to care for Gretchen since she lived downstairs. He and I both loved having them close to us. We worked very hard at not interfering in their lives, but it was nice to see them walking down the street together or sitting in our shared garden.

While Dan and Gretchen seemed to take it more in stride, John and I worried about the baby. I asked, "Gretchen, what exactly did the doctor say? On a scale of 1–10, how much should we worry?"

"As long as I stay off my feet, the doctor said I should be okay. They are worried the baby will come too soon, so I just need to stay still. It's preterm labor and lots of people get it."

"Will you let me know if anything happens, like if you start to bleed or feel pain?"

"Yes, I promise. Erica, it's going to be okay."

Dan left a cooler full of food by her bed each morning and hours' worth of "Sex and The City" tapes to watch. We bought her a nice chaise lounge chair so she could sit in the sun and read a book.

But John had other plans. He decided he would cook nice meals for their dinner. Gretchen's favorite became John's fried chicken, a recipe he stole from me. He worked in the garden, grocery shopped now for both families and cooked meals for Dan and Gretchen each night.

John and Gretchen had a special relationship. They were really good friends and anyone could tell they liked each other in addition to the familial relationship. They just enjoyed each other's sense of humor and liked talking to each other. John entertained her through those several months of bedrest during her first pregnancy.

John was in the hospital with Dan and Gretchen when Owen was born, while I was working in New York. It was John who fried chicken for her during bed rest, and according to Gretchen, "It was the best fried chicken ever."

John called me at my workplace in New York the morning of August 24, 2004. He gleefully told me, "Erica, I am in the hospital with Dan and Gretchen. The baby is coming today."

"No, the baby was supposed to wait for me to come home. I am so excited. Give me a blow by blow."

"Well, Dan is sitting next to Gretchen's bed. Gretchen is in labor, but not in a lot of pain yet."

"Aw, give them hugs for me. Tell them I love them."

"I am watching Gretchen's monitor. It really is amazing. I can tell on her monitor when she is going to have a contraction before she actually has one."

"How long do you think it's going to be?"

"I don't really know, but I will keep you posted. Uh oh, the doctor just came in and he told me it's time for me to leave the room now."

"Oh, my goodness! We are going to have our first grandchild."

"Here's my phone, say hello and good-bye to Gretchen and Dan."

"Thanks, John. Call me as soon as the baby is born. Do you think it's a boy or girl?"

"We will know soon enough. I love you, Sweets. Bye."

Owen Scott was born on August 24, 2004. Our first grandchild. His first home was in our garden apartment. We were like every other family going ga-ga over the newborn. The baby became our VIP. John and I walked Owen around our neighborhood in his stroller. We helped feed, bathe, change him and walk the floor when he was fussy. Gretchen was on maternity leave so she and John spent a lot of time together during the day taking care of Baby O.

Soon after Owen was born, Gretchen was shopping for birth announcements. She came home from shopping and told John, "I feel like I have a lump on my neck. What do you think it is?"

John replied, "I don't know, but you should probably get it looked at by a doctor."

The news came. Gretchen had thyroid cancer.

We were scared. We tried to remain calm. We were told some don't even think of thyroid cancer as cancer. We were told Gretchen needed to have her thyroid removed.

Surgery came and went. Baby Owen stayed with John and me overnight, so Dan could stand by Gretchen's side. Thankfully, it was a routine surgery, but she was left with a scar—one on her neck and one inside.

She thought, "What did this mean long term? Do I need to worry about my future?"

Gretchen was a mom now and she knew she was no longer living for just herself.

Gretchen and Dan had just bought a home in San Francisco and were preparing to move in just three months after Owen was born. Somehow that happened in the middle of thyroid cancer. Somehow Dan kept teaching school, I kept working, and John helped take care of the baby and Gretchen.

She needed to take radiation medication for a week to clear up any leftover cancer cells. I went with her to the hospital to get her pills. It was a strange and nerve-wracking task. We walked into the sterile hospital laboratory where she was given a container of a dangerous drug along with instructions on how to handle them and remain safe while she was on the regimen. She and I didn't talk to each other a lot about this, but we had to figure out how to take care of Baby O while she was in isolation. We were under stress but we just went into automatic "take care of stuff" mode.

Anyone near Gretchen could be exposed to radiation. Dan and Owen moved into our house and Gretchen stayed in her new home alone waiting for the radiation to wear off. We left food for her at her front door every morning. We waved at her from the car as she picked up her delivery.

Taking care of a three-month old baby meant night feedings, day feedings, diaper changing, walking the stroller and holding him when he cried. Our guest room now included a full-sized crib complete with a musical mobile, soft warm blankets, and stuffed animals. It felt natural to both John and me to return to parenting again. Natural and nice.

John and I stepped in to help so Dan could continue his teaching job. I knew it was really a struggle for the new mom and dad to have their life upended like this. They were supposed to be settling in with their new baby in their new house not adjusting to life with thyroid cancer- even for a short time. And, John and I wished for our son and daughter-in-law to have a carefree first born, first house, joyous experience.

Somehow it all ended. The radiation worked and we could all breathe again. We felt lucky when we learned no chemo was needed. Gretchen would take thyroid pills the rest of her life and have annual check-ups to monitor her endocrine system. But given what could've happened I think we all felt like we dodged a bullet.

A Promise Kept

Gretchen was well again and our lives could move on.

Backpacking

We stood next to the trailhead in Tuolumne Meadows with our loaded backpacks and our topographical map. I had twenty-five pounds while John carried close to forty each time we set out on an adventure. I always started with a bit of hesitance. *Can I make it*? I never wanted to do the same trail twice because then I would know what was in store for us. I liked the unknown.

This time we craned our necks to see Unicorn Peak at the top of the mountain, which designated where Nelson Lake sat. "Look, John. See that double peak at the top? We are going to climb way up there."

"Wow, Erica. That's going to be amazing. Can you imagine the views we'll see?"

"Oh my gosh, John. How high is that mountain? It looks higher than what we normally do."

"The trail book says it's ten thousand feet and a twenty-five-hundred-foot elevation change. We'll be okay. We can stop whenever you need a rest."

I led the way because John could see over me, but my view was hindered if he walked in front. As the trail widened, we walked side by side chatting about our kids, our jobs, the beauty of the forest, world politics, and whatever came to mind.

We broke our chatting with cherry-spitting contests. "Erica, see that tree up in front of us with the broken branches? Can you hit it with your cherry pit?"

"Ha, let's see. Oh my gosh, I almost got it. I can get you though. You are an easier target."

We exchanged cherry hits, staining each other's shirts with cherry juice. Laughing, we finally stopped and returned to just walking in silence for a bit.

We sang as we walked. For some reason, "Waltzing Matilda" was a favorite. Rarely did we encounter other hikers. We luxuriated in our togetherness. Sometimes John knew the names of the evergreen trees: Douglas Fir, Lodgepole Pine, Live Oak.

Slowly the flat land of the forest opened up to a climbing trail headed into the mountains. I knew this was when my soul would start to lift. My favorite part of hiking was always climbing granite rock. Getting above the tree line and looking around 360 degrees was something we didn't normally see. It was always thrilling. Unlike my everyday world, I could see it all in front of me. I was part of this that lay before me.

"Uh oh, John, there is snow all over this mountain. It's going to take forever to climb down.

"Oh, don't worry, Sweets. I have an idea. Pull out your air mattress. We'll slide down the mountain till we get to the next trail."

"Seriously?"

So, we laughed all the way down, put away our air mattresses and returned to granite.

We stopped on a flat rock. John pulled out the hard-boiled egg carrier and I reached in my bag for the peanut butter and jelly tubes and the bag of crackers.

After a bit, John asked, "Are you ready to get going again?"

"Can I have five more minutes?"

"Sure, I'm going over there behind that rock to take a leak."

"I'm jealous. It's so easy for you."

Finally, after hours of climbing and walking we were reaching the top. John made it first, but I was still a few climbing steps below the top. He reached down to grab my hand and pull me up. There we could stand on top and see the gorgeous, pristine, sparkling blue snow fed Nelson Lake, which was surrounded by the majestic Cathedral Range of the Sierras.

Breathtaking! John and I just stood in awe. I felt exhilarated, proud and euphoric when I made it to the top and John looked at me with a big smile on his face. "I love how you love Mother Nature," he told me.

Now, it was time to find our home for the next few days. I always wanted to take the first place where I could sit down, but John had other plans. He needed to explore the sites all around the lake to find the perfectly flat camp site. He wanted our sleeping bags to lie flat so his head was not below his feet or vice versa and there could not be rocks underneath our tent. So, I sat with our dumped backpacks while he circled the lake.

"Erica, I found a great spot. There's a lot of kindling near the site, flat ground under the trees and a short walk to the lake."

"Great, how far is it?"

"Not far. Just about half-way around."

"Okay, then, let's go. Come get your pack."

We had lots of jobs to do before we could relax. First, John made the bear bag. We took all our food and anything scented and threw it all into a big pillowcase. He tied a rope around the pillowcase with a rock at one end. Then the fun part was finding a branch high enough and stretched far enough out that would dissuade bears from climbing but low enough for him to reach with a good throw. The rope had to hang low enough for John to reach to pull down when we needed food. It was always a game.

Mama bears taught their babies to climb out onto branches to get backpackers' bear bags, so we had to find the kind of branch that would be hard for a baby bear to climb onto. In all the years we backpacked, the bears only won twice and they only ate all of our food once.

Once, I watched a bear come down from our bear bag tree with our pillow case. I just got very pissed as I stood on the ground in front of the tree and totally forgot any danger. Hands on my hips as I glared at the bear climbing down, I yelled, "Get out of here. Give me my stuff. Go, get out of here."

The bear ran and I chased him until he stopped and turned to look at me. *Uh oh, I thought. Now what have I done?*

I stopped and stood quietly with John coming up behind me. "What on earth are you doing, Erica?"

As the bear dropped our pillow-case and ran off, I said, "Well, he had our bear bag and all of our food." John just shook his head and hugged me.

Pitching the tent was a team effort. John laid out all the poles and the two of us attached the tent straps. Then he raised the tent while I breathed a sigh of relief. We swept the tarp that was our floor. It was my job to attach our sleeping bags to each other so we had a double bed. I placed the bags out neatly in the tent, put our clothes in pillow-cases to serve as lumpy headrests and threw blankets over the tops of the sleeping bags.

Together, we identified the area where our kitchen would be and found logs for our living room chairs. A fire pit sat in the center. We were now ready to sit back, relax and take in the view of our new homestead.

The morning started with John fishing and me jumping into the freezing, heart–stopping lake. John stood in admiration. The lake was filled with snow melt, but I needed my morning bath. I dove in, took a gasp of air, ducked my head in and climbed out as fast as I got in.

"Here, honey," John said as he handed me a towel. "I don't know how you do that."

John fished for trout so we did not have to eat dry food for dinner.

Meanwhile I found a nice sunny rock to use as my reading room. He loved fishing and I loved to eat his fish. Teamwork. He always gave me the fish cheeks. They were the sweetest part of the fish.

Backpacking with John was always so easy. He enjoyed doing all the hard work. He liked giving me time to relax and hang out while he cleaned the fish or made hash browns. We just fell into our routines. I watched our water jug to make sure I went to the lake to refill the jug. We hunted for kindling together.

Unspoken, we just knew how to be together in the wilderness.

One morning before breakfast, John said, "Let's explore a bit."

"Okay, should I bring water or food?"

"No, we will be right back."

We wandered cross country—off the trail as he liked—and after some time we were in a forest.

"John, it's getting hot and we don't have any water. I think we should go back to camp."

"Okay, head this way."

About an hour later I asked, "John, are we lost?"

"Do you mean now or forever?"

That became our inside joke. We used it over and over far into the future.

We took day hikes, made love on a rock, and talked. I read my book while he fished and I took photos while he took a nap in the shade. We owned the lake and the mountains around it.

Often, on our day hikes or just backpacking to our campsite we'd have to cross a stream. I was afraid of walking across logs especially if they were high off the ground. John helped me.

As he crossed the log to the other side he offered, "Erica, give me your pack. I'll carry it across for you."

"Are you sure you can do that, John? It's heavy."

"Yes, I'm sure. Just give it to me. Okay, now stand on the log and put one foot in front of the other. Take it slow. You are not going to fall."

As I gingerly crept across the log, one foot in front of the other, John came back from the other side to meet me halfway. He held his hand out. "Erica, grab my hand and walk slowly across the log."

I did it! I never fell in. This was our method for a long time, but each time I got braver and more sure of myself with John's help. And then one day, I no longer needed him to meet me halfway.

We loved the quiet, the beauty of our surroundings and just hanging out with Mother Nature.

John was our short-order cook, making breakfast on our small camp stove. Bacon and oatmeal. Hot chocolate or coffee. He even figured out how to toast bread on the little stove. He was the chef.

I washed the dishes.

Hiking out was different. Usually, it was downhill and faster. We knew the path and knew soon we would reenter civilization.

I, again, led the way. "Erica, heels first. That way you won't slip on the downhill slopes," he tutored me.

Daydreaming about real food after backpacking on a hot summer day was the best part of leaving.

"What do you want to eat or drink when we get out?" I asked.

"Oh, I want a nice, cold beer. What's your pleasure?"

"I think I want an ice cream cone. Chocolate."

We backpacked almost every weekend in the summers for years. We packed into Yosemite on every reasonable trail we could find. We traveled on trails through Carson Pass, Desolation Wilderness, Devils Postpile and Hetch Hetchy. One summer we packed the car to ascend the Grand Tetons in Wyoming for a different kind of adventure.

For the first time we headed out of state. A different mountain range. We needed to learn about the topography like the fact there was still ice among certain mountain trails. So, this was a first for both of us. We stayed in a motel the night before we began our ascent and looked up with awe as the spectacular Tetons loomed above us. It was a memorable trip for its beauty and adventure and loving companionship.

It was our thing.

We did it alone—just the two of us. It was ours to cherish. We both carried those memories forever.

The Peach Tree

The peach tree in our front yard gave birth to fully ripe, juicy, yellow-pink peaches every Fourth of July. This is exactly when John and I were in the Sierras. We went there every year on the Fourth. So, when we returned to San Jose from the wilderness, our front yard was carpeted with plump peaches we needed to rescue.

John picked up a peach and took a bite out of it as the juice dripped onto his dirty t-shirt. "Oh my god, Erica. This is delicious."

"I need to try one, I said." John leaned over and picked one up for me. We stood there with our backpacks on the ground and the car sitting in the driveway greedily enjoying the fruits of John's labor.

We had a small house with a small front yard in San Jose where I lived for eighteen years and John nine. He turned our front yard into a bountiful garden full of food I ate as I walked out our front door each morning on my way to work.

An apple tree, strawberries, squash, blackberries, tomatoes and our luscious peach tree surprised me each year with its gifts.

My absolute favorite was the peach tree. When I tried to make a crust from scratch it typically wound up on the kitchen wall. I am a good cook and a baker, but I cannot make a crust. John, on the other hand, was a crust–making specialist. His pie crusts were flaky, not too moist and definitely not too dry. I never knew his recipe for baking peach pie, because all I needed to know was that he was baking and I got to eat.

His pies were perfect. Just sweet enough and the peaches were not too hard or too soft. The big question was, "Would I add more calories to this sumptuous dessert by dishing out a scoop of cold vanilla ice cream onto the hot plate of peach pie?" Actually, it was never a real question.

John made peach daiquiris and sometimes we just enjoyed vanilla ice cream with sliced peaches while we read our books in bed.

On occasion, I baked peach cobbler which is so much easier and faster than peach pie, but also very tasty.

We shared our precious peaches and desserts with our friends who looked forward to our harvest. Everyone knew John's peaches were the summer's delight.

Those were good days. We were young and happy. We had full lives with our children, our friends and our work in our home that was not big or beautiful but filled with the generosity of love.

Love and Frustration

When we backpacked in our younger days, we went alone and did not want to share our experience, our joy, with anyone but each other. We had these memories to ourselves and they are so important. They brought us closer. They gave us a sense of how special our marriage and our love was. Not even Alzheimer's could break into our hearts—into our *EricaandJohn* space—and intrude on our love.

Our love is protected, safe and secure. Nothing breaks into our love. Our love belongs to us.

I wrote in my journal, *I notice John is changing. He is more in touch with his feelings. He talks to me more about how he feels - what he thinks. He is more affectionate. He is more frustrated and short-tempered. He is amped up and sometimes disconnected. But he is still John - funny, generous, smart, and interesting. He will always be the singular love of my life—regardless.*

One evening I was in the kitchen preparing dinner. Alexa was playing music—maybe Neil Diamond was on or the Bee Gees or Phantom of the Opera. John was in the back of the house watching TV. I was standing at the sink facing the windows to the outside world. Surprisingly, John walked up behind me, put his arms around my waist and pulled me close to him. He whispered, "I love you" and turned me around to dance to the music. John was not a dancer. I am. I shall remember the tender touch, the spontaneous affection and the feel of his arms holding me.

However, John became an impatient passenger in the car. I did most of the driving now. John could not handle the loss of control and commented negatively on my driving. He told me when to turn, when to pass, what lane to drive in, how fast or slow to go, and on and on. It made me really nervous when he yelled, "Watch out."

He was making me nuts. At one point, I stopped the car and I shouted at him, "John, I am going to have an accident. You are making me so nervous. You have to stop the commentary!"

He hung his head and uttered, "I'm sorry. I'll be quiet." Then I felt bad for making him feel bad. He stopped his insane backseat driving for a short time and then we had to have the discussion again.

"John, you can't keep telling me how to drive. I am going to have an accident." His anxiety and frustration overwhelmed him.

I thought about the things he has said—what he is thinking. Naturally, he was anxious.

John tells me he wants to die. He tells me he is in pain. He announces when he is having a good day or a bad day. He tells me he loves me and he worries about me. He worries about where I will live when he is no longer here. He worries that I won't have enough money or how I will take care of our big building. He worries that I will shut out our friends. He worries I will give up on life.

In spite of all this, somehow, we managed to laugh together and live our lives as though everything was normal. He worked in the garden. I worked on my photography. We came together around five in the evening for our ritual glass of wine, ate our dinner, watched some TV, and cuddled up together to sleep. We talked about the day's events, worried about politics, laughed at his jokes, and counted our blessings.

John talked to me about his future. In the beginning, we had no option but to live with Alzheimer's until the end—whenever that would be. He was so clear that he did not want to live beyond the time he was functional.

"Erica, I know you don't want to hear this, but we have to talk about it. We have to talk about what we will do when I can no longer take care of myself."

"John, there is nothing to talk about. I will take care of you. I will take care of you to the end. You are my husband and I love you."

"Honey, you know there will be a time when you won't be able to help me. I am too big and the whole thing will be too much for you."

"No, John. I will not let you go into an institution. Never! You will stay here with me. I will hire help if I have to, but I will not let you be put away."

"Sweets, you are not being realistic. I do not want to be a burden to you. I don't want to be a burden to anyone. If I can't be the master of my life, I want to die."

"I don't care if I am not being realistic." Sniffling. "I will never leave you in one of those places—without me. I will help you. I will find a way to help you. I promise."

Such hard conversations.

One weekend in February 2022 my sister, Judy, and brother-in-law, Keith, a doctor, visited from Wisconsin. Keith also spent time in the Air Force. So, both Keith and John had an expert's knowledge of guns.

We sat down in our cozy sunroom. John started a conversation with Keith about his illness.

Keith just said, "I'm so sorry, John. I am so sorry you have to go through this. I love you."

"Keith, I don't want to live when my brain doesn't work. My brain is my life. I don't want to sit in a chair, be a vegetable. That's not living. Can you give me some pills to end this when it's time?"

"No way. I am not going to jail for you. And Erica would go to jail as well. You can't get away with it. It's against the law for me to assist in a suicide. There would be an investigation and it is against the law to send medicine across state lines. I would be accused of being an accomplice to your death."

John accepted Keith's explanation and then asked, "Well, what is the best way to kill myself? What is the best way to do it with a gun?"

Keith went through all the body parts and explained the downside of each one. "There are just too many ways to mess up with a gun." He said. "The best way is to put the gun in your mouth and blow your brains out. It would be a mess for Erica to clean up." John and Keith discussed the pros and cons of hanging and poisoning yourself and finally John just said, " I had no idea it was that hard to kill yourself."

John suggested, "I could jump off the Golden Gate Bridge but that is not a for-sure thing, either."

The discussion lasted about an hour. I mostly listened and kept thinking, "I don't believe what I am hearing." It was the first of many bizarre conversations.

What was happening to us?

The Next Pregnancy

Right on plan, Gretchen became pregnant again. The two kids would be 26 months apart. By this time, Gretchen was working for me as a moderator at Baccus Research, so I saw her every day that I was in town. I could watch her tummy grow and see when she got tired. I could insist she should go home at a decent hour. I listened to her complain about the Chinese sauces being made downstairs that made her nauseous once a week. It was altogether lovely.

Gretchen had been working for ad agencies in San Francisco and spent crazy long hours in the office. She spent a lot of time miserable and I used to tell her, "Gretchen, anytime you need a job, you can come work for me." In 2003, she and Dan were engaged and both John and I were ecstatic. I answered the phone one afternoon in my office and heard Gretchen crying, "I can't do this anymore. Did you mean it when you said I could work for you?"

"Hang up the phone, quit your job, and come to work for me tomorrow."

Sniffling, she said, "Thank you."

Her story later on was that she needed to plan their wedding and she had no time to do it at the job she had. She knew that I would give her that time, so she called me to ask for a job. She was right. Of course I would.

But it was more than that. She learned a whole new career and was really good at moderating. I trained her on every aspect of the business and she became my All Star. Eighteen years later, Gretchen is still working as a market research moderator.

In October 2006, I was in Dallas preparing to conduct focus groups for Dell, one of my favorite clients. I was sitting in an office area talking to my client. Someone said, "Erica, you have a phone call."

I took the phone. It was Gretchen. In a controlled and somber voice, she explained, "Erica, I have bad news. I have cancer again. It is some kind of lymphoma." As I listened, I became terrified. She was nine months pregnant. This was blood cancer. She went on, "They are going to take the baby tonight—they are going to induce labor. They say I need to start chemo as fast as possible, so they want to deliver the baby today. They don't want to wait."

I hung up the phone shaking. Barry, my client, asked, "What's wrong, Erica?" I explained and he said, "I'm going to call a cab to take you to the airport. I am going to get you airline reservations now. You need to go home."

"What about the focus groups, Barry?"

"Don't worry about the focus groups, I'll do them."

Choking back tears, I said, "Thank you, Barry." I thought about Gretchen and my son and my new grandchild and worried about what would happen. I was petrified and I knew Dan and Gretchen were very frightened.

I arrived at the hospital in time to be in the delivery room before she gave birth. John was at home with Owen. At that moment, all I wanted was for a healthy baby to be born and for Dan and Gretchen to put aside their impending disaster and enjoy the birth of their baby.

Noah James was born October 17, 2006. Healthy, squirmy and pink.

Gretchen was allowed to return home for one week. She had one week to spend with her two boys. She had one week to feed her baby and change his diapers and hold him close. She had one week to cuddle two-year-old Owen and give him her love.

Then, life completely changed. Gretchen returned to the hospital. The doctors identified her cancer as Burkitt's Lymphoma, an aggressive form of blood cancer. The upside was that it was supposed to respond to treatment well. Gretchen spent the next six months of her life in a fetal position in the hospital. In and out of ICU, close to death, she fought to stay alive for her children.

She won.

During that time Gretchen's mom, who lived in Hong Kong, came to stay at Gretchen and Dan's house. Dan asked her to take care of Noah, while John and I would care for Owen. John took the day shift and because I was still working, I took the evening shift: dinner, bath, story time, and sleep. Dan continued his teaching job, visited Gretchen in the hospital and spent as much time as he could with his two sons.

It took all of us to take care of the two babies and visit Gretchen. The stress and fear sat in our hearts. Taking care of Owen was a bright light in our day and helped John and I manage our emotions.

John and I shut our lives down for the six months of lymphoma. We put our social life on hold and dedicated ourselves to helping Gretchen and her family. John and I did not have to discuss this. We both understood this was what we needed and wanted to do.

Perhaps understandably, I destroyed John's van in the UCSF parking garage. The slots were too narrow and it was really hard to back a big car out with tears clouding my eyes. It seemed like every time I visited Gretchen, I made another dent in the car. I didn't care. Neither did John.

Visiting Gretchen was an act of futility. She was too sick to sit up in bed or hold a conversation. Owen was not allowed to visit because her immune system was drastically compromised and he was a two-year-old full of germs.

But one day, the doctors deemed it possible for Owen to visit. A special area was set up for Gretchen away from visitors where Owen could see his mommy for a short time. John was not in favor of the visit. He worried that seeing Gretchen with tubes, bald head and skinny body would scare him. But John and I were hopeful and took Owen to see his mommy.

It was not a good visit. Gretchen became very tired and Owen really didn't know how to react. John was right. We should have waited.

It was Gretchen's birthday and I wanted to do something special for her. She loves cheesecake. It is her favorite dessert. I decided I would bake a cheesecake for her and bring it to the hospital. Not only had she zero interest in eating cake, she had to be taken to the ICU abruptly while I was sitting in a chair by her bedside. I left feeling bereft and scared. I offered the cheesecake to the nurses and prayed to the universe to make her well again. It was a dumb thing to bring cake to Gretchen, who was so sick. Eating was the last thing on her mind. I guess I was trying to do something normal.

It was during this time that John seriously bonded with Owen. I have images in my head of the two of them cuddling so hard and giggling like crazy. It was during this time, John walked like Forrest Gump around San Francisco with Owen on his shoulders, played trains in the upstairs playroom, laid down on the floor holding Owen high above his head as he flew in the sky or sat him on his lap shaking like an earthquake.

John was a rock. He helped Owen by playing with him and keeping his life normal during the day. He kept his positive spirit and encouraged me to follow suit so Owen would not feel frightened.

Owen spent a lot of afternoons and nights with us at our house. Here he could cuddle with us in our bed if he felt lonely and he could run through all the rooms in our house chasing John and never catching him. Here he could watch old Disney videos and belly-laugh at Tom and Jerry's antics or Popeye the Sailor Man. Here he could help me bake cookies and make a mess in the kitchen painting with watercolors. Here he could have fun, feel loved and safe away from cancer.

Somehow, we all made it through those six months. Gretchen came home to be a mommy and eventually she returned to work. Slowly normal life resumed.

The Move

Sometimes life is full of irony. One Saturday morning I joined Danny and Owen at My Gym. It's a wonderful place full of little kids who climb and jump and run and do gym kind of things like swinging from the rafters and crawling across barrels with a teacher. I loved going along to watch.

While we had our eyes on Owen, who at six years old was somewhat shy but very ready to take a tumble with the other kids, Danny said to me, "Mom, I need to tell you something."

"Uh oh," I thought. "That kind of thing never sounds like good news."

"Gretchen and I have been talking about a lot of things. I know you are going to be upset, but I need you to understand. We are moving to Chicago."

Choking back my hysteria, I asked all the questions, "But why? When? Will you change your mind?"

Dan was so smart to pick a public place to tell me. I could not create a disturbance.

I kept thinking about how I brought Danny to California when he was six. It was a good move for him. He thrived in the sunshine and the climate was healthy for his asthma. He loved to play soccer year-round and ski with me in the winter. He was happy in California. Now his life choices led him to return to the very place he and I left.

I dreaded telling John. I knew how disappointed he would be. But I had no choice.

"John, I have some bad news. Sit down so we can talk about it."

"Is everyone okay?"

"Yes, but Gretchen and Danny have decided to move back to Chicago."

"WHAT? WHY?"

"Well, you know Gretchen has a big family back there and Kristine has 3 kids. Gretchen wants the 5 cousins to grow up close to each other. She wants to be near her family."

"What are we—chopped liver?"

"Look, you know this isn't you alone. I'm a mess. We will just have to figure it out so we maintain our relationship with the boys. Let's not make it harder for us or them. But I know how you feel. I said the same thing to Danny."

In June of 2011, they moved to the suburbs of Chicago. Kyle had already moved to the suburbs of Kansas, so now all of our grandkids would be long-distance.

And so, our lives changed. I retired in January 2011, so I was free to travel with John. We prioritized family and learned how to make long distance work. Dan and Gretchen promised that our annual Tahoe summer vacation would continue as would a ski trip each spring. With those traditions holding ground, we made new ones.

October: The boys had a Columbus Day break at school that conveniently arrived near Noah's birthday. We flew to their home each year.

November/December. Thanksgiving and Christmas. We celebrated at least one holiday together.

February. President's Day offered up another chance for a long weekend for us with the boys.

March. Ski trip, first in Tahoe and then one year the snow was much better in Colorado so we began the tradition of meeting in Denver for a spring break Colorado ski trip.

June: Dan and Gretchen sent the boys to California to spend a week with us. When they were too young to fly alone, I flew there to pick them up.

August. Our annual Tahoe family week together.

Then we started all over again. It worked. John and I talked to the boys on the phone every possible Sunday. It was part of our ritual to be a part of their lives and to know them not as strangers but as people. I still talk to each of them every Sunday.

Our camping tradition began with their visit each June. Kiera and

Taryn, who lived in California, joined our little camping family every year. For years we took the 4 kids all over California to camp in the redwoods, by a river, at the ocean, or on a mountain.

They ate Papa's amazing bacon and hash browns in the morning, learned how to round up kindling wood for the night time bonfire, slept in tents listening to the sounds of animals all around each evening and the birds in the morning. Papa told stories and helped them put bait on their fish hooks.

One of Noah's favorite stories still makes him laugh today.

Papa started with, "Once upon a time there was a little boy who slept soundly. While he was sleeping little tiny people made from lint in the boy's pocket climbed out of his pocket and slid down the little boy's nose. They were very little so they did not wake up the little boy.

"The lint people hosted nose sliding competitions to see who could ride the furthest. Some of the lint people were very scared. At the end of the competition whoever was able to slide off of the boy's nose and travel the furthest was declared the winner. It was sort of like ski jumping.

The winner won the right to collect the lint from the little boy's belly button."

Each year was different, but each year sealed us in a new memory and coated us with love.

Papa John

John was the kind of Papa who purposely put Owen's boots on when it was raining and took him outside to jump in the puddles. Mud mattered not. He carried Owen on his shoulders everywhere they walked.

"I can't talk to him if he's in a stroller. He's too far away from me with his back to me."

John pointed out the flowers and asked Owen to say the word, or truck when they saw one in the street or clouds when they looked up. I think Owen learned to talk on John's shoulders.

He carried Owen all over the neighborhood ducking under trees or letting Owen reach for the leaves to find out how they felt or smelled. Riding on the J-Train and getting off at Mission Dolores Park to run around on the grass was a favorite.

He played Marco Polo in the pool with Drew and Haley, Kyle's kids, long after any reasonable adult could stand it. He easily wore a dinosaur head to play pretend with Haley and flew drone planes and fished in the lake with Drew. Nothing was too silly or too boring or too tiring. John was all in.

He taught both Owen and Noah how to have a legitimate sock fight—one that I would not let him do when Dan and Kyle were young. Now, with grandchildren, I didn't care if a vase was broken. John took all his socks out of the drawer, rolled them up tight and then he hid behind the bed or the sofa or a chair. The boys took the other side of the room. With the socks shared between the two teams, they threw them at each other as hard as they could. Socks went everywhere along with the sounds of the giggles and screams.

John wrestled and ran races, put their t-shirts on backwards because he didn't care about doing it the right way, and slid down slides when he could fit. He fed them ice cream and peanut butter sandwiches and chose bedtime to wrap them up in a towel like a burrito and throw them onto the bed.

Together we took them to the beach and buried them in the sand. John hunted for sand crabs and rolli-pollies with them, taught them about the currents, and helped them jump the waves in the ocean. They collected rocks together. I still have some on my shelf. The most fun was taking them home and hosing them off with cold water in the backyard before they could carry their sand-infested bodies into our house.

We took Owen camping when Noah, at one-year-old, was too young to join us. Owen was three. He learned to find a pee tree, curl up in a sleeping bag in a tent and collect sticks to make a campfire. We took Owen and Noah camping every summer for the next fourteen years.

We were a bit worried about Owen's first trip—worried he might be afraid to sleep in a tent in the dark. We had Plan B. Friends lived near our campsite, so we asked if we could spend the night in case the dark tent was too much for Owen. Sure enough, Owen loved the tent as long as it was light outside. Dusk came and Owen popped his head out of the tent to tell us, "It's time to go home now. I don't want to sleep here."

I comforted him. "Owen, honey, we can go sleep at Jim and Jean's house and come back in the morning for more fun."

"Yes," Papa said. "We will make bacon on the stove and drink hot chocolate."

So, Plan B went into action. We packed up our sleeping bags, slept at Jean's house and returned to our campsite for breakfast.

John was the one who started the flashlight tag tradition when we went camping. He gathered all the kids he could find in the campgrounds and got a good game going. He built bows and arrows, slingshots, fishing poles and toy boats for the kids for our outdoor adventures.

When Owen was three, he told Papa, "I want to build a sailboat and I know exactly what it will look like." He described the boat in detail to Papa, who drew the picture to make sure it fit Owen's imagination. Once Owen approved the drawing, the two went into our garage and Owen built his first of many toys with Papa.

Papa never said, "No." He always had an idea for fun. He was a kid too who wanted to play, forget the rules and create an adventure to remember.

loved the tent as long as it was light outside. Dusk came and Owen popped his head out of the tent to tell us, "It's time to go home now. I don't want to sleep here."

I comforted him. "Owen, honey, we can go sleep at Jim and Jean's house and come back in the morning for more fun."

"Yes," Papa said. "We will make bacon on the stove and drink hot chocolate."

So, Plan B went into action. We packed up our sleeping bags, slept at Jean's house and returned to our campsite for breakfast.

John was the one who started the flashlight tag tradition when we went camping. He gathered all the kids he could find in the campgrounds and got a good game going. He built bows and arrows, slingshots, fishing poles and toy boats for the kids for our outdoor adventures.

When Owen was three, he told Papa, "I want to build a sailboat and I know exactly what it will look like." He described the boat in detail to Papa, who drew the picture to make sure it fit Owen's imagination. Once Owen approved the drawing, the two went into our garage and Owen built his first of many toys with Papa.

Papa never said, "No." He always had an idea for fun. He was a kid too who wanted to play, forget the rules and create an adventure to remember.

The Caretaker

John was not really a caretaker, at least not one typically imagines. He was solely motivated by his desire to help people. He wasn't interested in medical specifics or cures. He wanted to be the good guy and he understood sometimes he was really needed.

I have had five joint replacements over the last twenty years. John instinctively knew how to make me comfortable through two hip replacements. He knew just how to place the pillow under my leg so I could sleep, and he knew when to let me do it on my own. My shoulder replacements were more complicated. There were three of those because my right shoulder had to be operated on twice. Not having the use of my dominant right hand or arm for three months is tough.

"John, can you blow-dry my hair?"

"Okay, tell me what to do."

My hair just hit my shoulders for my first two replacements. When my left shoulder needed replacement, I had long COVID hair which turned out to be easier to manage.

"Take the big round brush in your right hand and the hair dryer

A Promise Kept

in your left. Curl the hair around the brush and blow it dry. Do it in layers and start with the hair underneath."

"Okay, let's give it a try."

John was so talented with his hands that he got quite good at styling my hair. We shared some laughs as he was learning, but he was so patient. He was way more patient with me than I was with him.

My friends complimented me on my hair during the time he was my hairstylist. They were amazed when I told them John was "doing" my hair.

"John's blow-drying your hair?" Cheryl asked in amazement. You gotta be kidding! No way could Tom do mine."

Not having the use of my right hand meant it was hard to cook, so I stood next to him in the kitchen and directed him so he could make certain recipes. John was a pretty good cook as long as he made his things: fish, eggs of any kind, French toast, bacon and grilled cheese sandwiches.

I was the one who got sick every now and then. I had been hospitalized several times over the years for acute curable illnesses. I can count the number of times John even had a cold in the forty-one years we were married. He brought tea and toast to my bed, ran to the drugstore to buy a new thermometer because we kept losing the old one, and picked up prescriptions for me. He covered me with blankets when I had chills and tried to keep me comfortable.

I have never been comfortable being comforted, but he made it easy for me to accept his kindness.

If someone was detained on the roadside, John had to stop to offer his help. If someone fell down, John was the first one to offer his hand. My daughter-in-law and sister-in-law used to greet John at the door with a "honey-do" list. He loved helping them. He felt needed and appreciated.

At least twice yearly we visited my brother and sister-in-law in Utah where they lived with their three kids. Each time Louise greeted us at the door with a big smile on her face. "Hi, guys. I missed you both, but, John, I missed you more."

John laughed and said, "Hey, Louise. Give me a hug. What's up?"

"You can come in and relax, but my toolbox is ready for you whenever you are ready."

"Sure, you know I am happy to help. Do you have a list for me?"

My single friends knew they could ask John for help. One time a friend and neighbor asked John to help her hang her new curtains and another friend called sobbing one day when she found her cat dead in her yard. She wanted John to come over to help her with her cat. John helped friends build houses and plant gardens.

He was also very free with advice. I often said to him, "John, be careful with what you advise. People listen to you." He gave counsel on business decisions, affairs of the heart and life's choices. Kyle and John discussed Kyle's entrepreneurial businesses on the phone and I often heard John recommending "what to do." Or he'd advise Anne, our single young friend, and tell her to "dump him or not."

He just thought he could offer what he thought, and people could make up their own minds. I used to worry he overstepped.

A Promise Kept

Kyle recently said to me, "When I have a question about my business, the first thing I think is I need to call Dad. And now Dad is not here. I don't have anyone to talk things over with."

Tomatoes

He stood in the greenhouse, paintbrush in hand, readying himself to be the bee.

Buzz, buzz, buzz.

"I carefully touch the bristles to the pollen-filled pestle and brush it onto the flower's leaf," he explained to me. You have to be the pollinator every day when I am gone. Bees can't get into the greenhouse."

Each flower on each plant was exquisitely tended. John made his way to his house of tomatoes every morning. Each day he considered the need for water or debugging a plant.

Would I have the patience to do this?

As spring turned into summer, John reported, "The tomatoes are growing. They are the size of a small tennis ball now." Or he'd plead, "Come look, Erica, your tomatoes are growing."

Or, "Wow, there are some yellow ones mixed in with the reds."

As days passed, finally John climbed our thirty-two stairs to our kitchen and plunked down a handful of juicy, ripe, mostly very red tomatoes just for me. I sliced one, not too thick, not too thin, slowly, seasoned it with kosher salt and took my first luscious bite of the summer. The sweet juice slid down my throat and I turned to John, "Thank you. These are awesome. I love you."

The tomatoes were a first sign of summer days where John and I sat on the patio admiring his garden and enjoying our time together.

Sharing The News

It was June 2021 when we finally told our older grandchildren, nieces and nephews about John's disease. We decided we had to tell our closer family, but we would do it on an as-needed basis. First, we told Danny, Gretchen, Kyle and Lori. Judy and Keith were also the first to know. Later on, we had to choose a time to tell our sisters-in-law and nieces and nephews. As we told each group, it became more real that John truly had an incurable disease.

I still spent a lot of time thinking we were pretty okay. I began to adjust to John's changes and it all didn't seem so bad. I didn't mind repeating something dozens of times in a row. I didn't mind reminding him his golf date was at Indian Valley at 10:10 that Thursday. Denial crept into my thinking. It allowed me to relax a bit even though it was a temporary relief. In the first year, these forgotten pieces of information seemed minor to me. We still spooned at night, laughed with each other, watched the Warriors win and lose basketball games, and we still held hands walking to Chestnut Street.

I started to adapt to John's memory losses. I started to anticipate what he needed to function so he wouldn't need to ask me. I started to think we were normal. I started to forget how active John once was. I started to forget how independent and capable

John always was. I started to forget John's love for arguing for argument's sake as he became more passive and less engaged. I started to think his dependence on me was acceptable to him and to me.

When John worked in the garden, I began to go down there around 1 PM and bring him a sandwich.

"John, you haven't eaten all day."

"I'm not hungry."

"John, you have to eat. Please. It doesn't matter if you are hungry. Please eat something."

He pleaded, "Just let me finish pruning this tree."

"Okay, I'll wait and sit with you."

We used to walk down to the Golden Gate Bridge often or bike across the bridge to Tiburon. We both loved the exercise and the beauty of our surroundings.

I'd ask John, "Hey, do you want to get up tomorrow morning and walk to the Bridge?"

"Well, maybe, let's see how I feel in the morning."

I'd cajole, "It will be good for you. It would be fun. We can walk as far as you want and turn around. We don't have to go all the way."

John couldn't commit. "I don't know, Erica."

I learned to have patience while repeating the most mundane news. This conversation would be had many times during the day and it became normal to me.

John: Erica, what's happening tonight?

Erica: We are going out to dinner with Cheryl and Tom at 7 p.m.

John: What do I have to wear?

Erica: Just clean jeans and shirt.

John: What time are we going?

Erica: We need to be there at seven.

We were not telling most of our friends. At first, I did not want our friends to see John differently. But mostly, I didn't want to open us both up to friendly advice, offerings of books to read, research to consult, and all the stuff well-meaning friends think will help. As John was the patient and I the "caretaker" (God, how I hate that word) it was confusing enough and concerning enough to just ingest the medical information from the UCSF neurology and palliative care teams. We did not want or need amateur popular advice from outside the medical arena.

I did read some Harvard research on Alzheimer's and nutrition. I bought a lot of blueberries. It became my joke with John: "Put blueberries in your Cheerios and your memory will be fine."

I believed in the medical industry. I came from a family of doctors; my dad was an anesthesiologist, my uncle was an internist, my older brother was a pediatric cardiologist, my sister is a nurse, her husband is an emergency medicine doctor, one of my sisters-in-law was a medical technician and my younger brother was a PhD psychologist. One can only imagine the dinner table conversations.

When I was in college my dad took me into the operating room one day and let me stand at the patients' heads while he administered the anesthesia. I observed five operations that day—and one was a C-section. That was pretty awesome.

I am not a person who believes alternatives to traditional medicine work. I believe in science. I also believe in UCSF, one of the finest hospital systems in the country. This is all to say my heart and mind were going to follow the advice of John's doctors. I trusted them and thought if anything new appeared in the medical market, the UCSF physicians would be aware of it.

"God, I hate hospitals. I hate doctors and I really don't like going to UCSF," John complained to me one day as we were driving to a neurology appointment.

I pleaded, "But John, they are only trying to help you. With this disease, what options do we have? We need these people."

And John argued back, "But Erica, the end is going to be the same regardless. There is no cure. There is no remedy. I am going to lose my person and I'm going to die. I will take the pills for you, but they are doing nothing for me." He was frustrated, but I knew he was also a realist.

With his answer clear in my heart, I held in my tears, took a deep breath and smiled at him.

As John's memory loss became more apparent, we had to acknowledge his illness. Telling people was another step in the progression of the disease—another change in our lives that said the end was nearing.

Making the decision to tell people was difficult enough, but then we had to decide who to tell and how to share the news. It felt like we were making more and more decisions that we had never considered before. Our conversations were becoming weird.

"Erica, I do not want to spend years sitting in a chair, drooling, and looking out a window."

"John, honey, I promise you we will figure something out. I also promise you that you will always stay here with me."

"That is not realistic, Erica."

"I don't care if it is realistic. I will not put you away somewhere. You will be with me."

June 2021: Email to Extended Family

Hello Everyone,

It is time for me to share some information with you. I shall try to be as objective as I can. Because you all are so important to John and me and so loved by both of us, I believe it is time to tell you that John was diagnosed with Alzheimer's in January 2020. For a while, there were very few noticeable symptoms, but now, if you spend time with John, you are likely to become aware of his forgetfulness. He has trouble remembering new information.

I want to emphasize that he is still the same Uncle John Beard. He is still loving and kind, funny and generous, and smart. I am telling you all about this now so you have choices about how you spend time with him. You all have lovely young lives you are living and are appropriately busy, so no one is expecting you to do anything out of the ordinary. We have been so fortunate to have close relationships with all of you and just a few weeks ago we had a great time with you, Ted, and your family as well as with you, Trevor, and Aparna.

You can ask me any questions you want, but I will tell you now I probably don't have any answers. This disease is different for everyone. It progresses differently and shows itself differently. We are living with gratitude for each lovely day we have with each other and with our friends and family.

Dan, Kyle, Lori, Judy, Keith and Louise have known for sometime now. We just told Owen and Noah during our visit to Chicago—Owen asked if Papa had Alzheimer's so we knew it was time to tell them.

We are taking a family trip with Dan's family and Kyle's family this August to Hawaii and in September John and I are going to Europe. We are taking advantage of time. So, there it is. We are aging and nothing is supposed to stay the same.

Love to you all.

"Auntie", Erica

Erica Baccus

Responses from nieces and nephews:

Dear Erica,

First off, I'm sorry I didn't respond sooner. I'm not quite sure what to say except that anything I can say seems inadequate to express both how sorry I am to hear about John's diagnosis as well as how important both he and you have been in my life.

Trevor, Lauren and myself were lucky to have a very charmed childhood. We have too many good memories from when we were kids to count. You and John are central to so many of those memories. Going out to visit you guys, having Christmas in Utah or in SF, Christmas in Tahoe—I'm not sure if this is typical in other families but I know I was always excited to see my aunt and uncle. I can't imagine having a more loving and fun aunt and uncle than you and John. I hope Sylvia and I can be half the aunt and uncle to our future nieces/nephews that you and John are to us.

I can't imagine how scary it must be looking towards the future and not being sure about what it holds for you. But I hope you know that no matter what, you will always be an important part of our lives, that we care about you and love you, and that we will always be excited to see Aunt Erica and Uncle John for as long as we can. I say we because I know Trevor and Lauren feel the same as I do about you and John.

I'm writing John a letter that I'll send so you don't need to show him this email, I just wanted to tell you that I love you and will be thinking about you guys. I hope for the best and will cherish whatever time left we have with John.

Love, Alex

A Promise Kept

Auntie Erica,

I JUST read your email and I really don't know what to say.

We love u guys and I believe that the disease will not be easy on John, my favorite American uncle.

I know we live on the other side of the world but I want you to know we are here for you.

I was worried about John's health when we were in Santa Cruz, but just because you were so worried about him finding his way back to the beach.

John is VERY lucky to have you on his side. I am so sad we live so far away and missed/ are still missing all of you guys. We just have to do better about visiting.

I love you, Agata

PS. I hope my English makes sense.

Hi Erica,

Thank you for sharing this with us. I can't imagine how hard the diagnosis was to receive, or how tough it is for you to talk about it. John is one of the kindest, most welcoming people I've ever met. I'm so glad that we could spend time with you both when you were here to visit. More than that, we're so glad that you and John could celebrate our wedding with us—it truly would not have been the same without you both there.

At the moment, we are planning to come back out to CA in mid-July, and would love to see you both while we're in town (if you're not traveling then!). We'll let you know as soon as we make our plans concrete. Otherwise, whenever you both have time, we always enjoy zoom calls!

All our love,

Aparna & Trevor

Our family was wonderful. Each person just said, "Whatever you need, we are here to help. What can we do? We love you."

What more could John and I ask for?

Our nephews lived close by so they could spend more time with John than normal. But our children and grandchildren were out of state so our lives continued with them as it always had. Throughout the years that John and I knew he was sick, we never changed anything in our lives.

Since Dan and his family lived in the suburbs of Chicago, Kyle and his family lived outside of Kansas City and Lori, John's stepdaughter (more a daughter though), lived in Sacramento, the distance from us did not allow them to see John's decline.

They were constantly telling me on the phone, "He seems normal to me." Even after visiting with us, Dan or Kyle, or somebody would tell me, "Mom, John seems like John. He hasn't really changed much."

Sometimes I let the comment go. Sometimes I'd say, "You don't see what I see." Or maybe I asked, "What are you trying to tell me? That he really doesn't have Alzheimer's?"

I understood this made them feel better. I knew they believed the diagnosis, but they could not see the changes I saw and John felt. It was true that one could have a conversation with John and not notice he was making stuff up, because he couldn't remember what actually happened. I knew, though. Denying his changes helped them to not worry. But it made me feel like I was so alone in this mess. I felt my worries were totally invalidated. They were trying to make me feel less concerned, but instead I felt like I had no one to turn to except my sister and brother-in-law who were both medical professionals who understood exactly what was happening.

Judy and Keith became my go-to people for Alzheimer's information, consoling, and understanding. I had my cell phone in my hand. Judy answered hers. "Hi Erica."

I cried and cried and cried. I could not speak. She simply listened. I said, "I am sorry. I just need to talk. John forgot how to get to the golf course today. He had left to play with his Thursday buddies and after about 20 minutes he walked into the house. I asked, "John, what are you doing here?"

He calmly answered, "I couldn't find the right turn-off. It was getting too late to go, so I came home."

Choking back more tears, I sputtered out, "That's another first." Judy just listened and said, "I am sorry, Erica. I am so sorry. Do you want to talk to Keith?" "No," I said, "It's okay. There is nothing he can do."

Sometimes I called Keith and asked, "Why is John sleeping so much? Should I try to keep him awake and more active?"

Keith always explained medical issues in lay terms so I could understand. He simply said, "Erica, John's brain is slowing down. His brain is in charge of everything so as the disease progresses, he will be more tired—more sleepy. I am so sorry, Erica. I am so sorry you and John have to go through this."

As time passed and we finally told friends, they too often said, "John seems fine." or "John seems normal."

I felt crazy. What I knew about John was denied by most everyone except Judy and Keith and the doctors. John worked hard at looking normal.

I felt like I was living in an alternate reality. Either John's illness existed or it didn't. How could I tread both worlds sanely?

With a disease like Alzheimer's which can progress at various speeds, people are confused about what they think they should see. John never forgot anyone's name, and he never lost his vocabulary. Yes, he repeated himself continuously and sometimes lost his way driving, and, in the end, became delusional, but a casual friendly dinner out with John remained pretty constant over time. Friends were aware he had a disease, but they had no idea how serious it was.

I was alone in this.

When we told our closest friends, they were supportive in their best ways even though they could not truly understand how the disease affected both of us. It surprised me that they instinctively knew how to handle situations. No one made a big deal of it.

In September 2021 we were in Italy with a large group of friends sharing a beautiful large estate in Tuscany. When John couldn't find his room and wandered into someone else's room, Lisa just casually pointed him in the right direction. She told me, "Erica, I found John wandering around in our wing. He was looking for your bedroom, so I told him which way to go. I hope that was okay." Our friends contributed to his well-being.

"That's fine, Lisa. Thank you."

When John played golf with a group, Tom asked John. "Hey John, why don't you ride with me? I'll drive the cart."

But what they didn't see was what I saw. John had an amazing capacity for keeping up the show of "being fine" with a little memory loss. What I saw was my husband shedding all that made him himself and I did not wish to ruin John's show. The truth was that both John and I knew what was really happening.

Below is a letter I wrote to my good friend, Cheryl. I tried explaining what our lives were like and why we needed privacy. I do not think I succeeded in either endeavor, but I tried.

2020

Hi Cheryl,

I feel the need to say a few things since our talk earlier today about John. It is really difficult for me to discuss John's situation with anyone. What is going on with John for him personally and how it impacts me and our marriage is extremely personal to me. I have confided in a very few people as I mentioned to you.

Perhaps there will be a day down the road when I will need to let people know what is happening, but right now I do not want people to look at John differently or treat him differently. I also don't want our lives to be the topic of idle conversations.

John is a sensitive and caring man who is generous with his love for his friends and family. So, I am trying to protect those relationships. And yes, I know he has told several people but he does not remember who he has told. John feels close to Tom and I think it is a good thing that Tom can talk with John either in a joking manner about memory difficulties or seriously. But that is between John and Tom.

To be very candid with you, I figure John and I have about five good years left together. Hopefully, I am totally wrong. We are both trying very hard to live one day at a time and appreciate the goodness of each day. Actually, this situation is one of the reasons I feel it is important for us to risk flying to Chicago for Xmas.

I am sure you know John and I have had an amazing marriage for the last thirty-eight years and I am forever grateful for his love and friendship. We find humor in our lives today and continue to live a normal life. With that said, I know I am learning new lessons each day about patience and kindness and shall need to keep on learning. I will be there for him as he has been there for me so many times. That is marriage.

I guess I am writing all this because I felt the need to explain a bit. Thanks for listening.

Your friend, Erica

As John's disease continued to progress, we decided we needed to communicate with the family to make sure their needs were addressed. I arranged monthly Zoom meetings with Lori and Kyle and with Dan and Gretchen and Judy and Keith. The purpose of the meetings was to let our family who lived out of state understand how John was doing—what were his symptoms, what did doctors say, and to answer any questions they may have had. John participated in these meetings, so nothing was a secret. Judy and Keith helped answer medical questions.

Below is an agenda I wrote for a meeting we had on May 12, 2022.

I. How do we schedule these meetings so everyone can join?

II. Status

    A. EEG—myoclonus and energy

    B. Lack of energy

    C. Memory is part of our lives now

    D. I'm afraid to let John go by himself to buy beer at the baseball game

    E. I'm doing the finances now

    F. John doesn't really initiate conversations with me

    G. The Apple watch was a good idea

III. What do we need?

    A. Judy & Keith's visit was good.

B. Get Keith's reactions

C. Maybe Dan and Kyle could visit regularly

IV. Questions

A. Changes to our health care directive

B. Get DNR bracelet for John and ask doctor to make DNR an official status

We also set up routine Zoom poker games which we started playing during COVID. It was a fun way for the family to stay in touch with John, and taking John's money was a little extra treat.

I started the games: "Hi guys. You are all looking good. We are still waiting for Trevor to check in."

John: "Hi everyone. Ready to lose your money?"

Gretchen: "I've got my $20 ready and I am happy to take more from you all."

Owen: "What are we playing tonight? I've got my poker face ready."

John remained constant in his ability to play poker to the end.

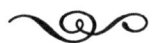

2022: A Turning Point

We played golf together throughout our marriage. We had so much fun trying out different courses whenever we went on a trip somewhere, and we played on home courses many weekends either with friends or just the two of us. It was a social thing. Playing with John was like taking a beautiful walk in the park with your best friend. About the 15th hole I started to think about where we might have dinner and a nice glass of wine. We were both hackers, but John was a better hacker than me. John had a keen eye for the technical side of golf.

"John, help me. I keep hitting the top of the ball. I don't know why."

"Take a practice swing and let me see. Oh, you're too far from the ball, Erica. Just move closer—just an inch."

"Okay, let's see what happens." I swung and hit the ball a mile. "Thanks, honey. Next time you can tell me if you see something wrong."

He and I kept playing. Only close to the end it was different. He wanted to drive the cart and keep score as always. His memory lapses made it hard for him to keep track.

"John, go back. You passed my ball way back."

"Oh, sorry. I forgot about your ball."

"John, slow down. I am going to fall out of the cart. Did you put our scores down? I don't see anything for the last two holes."

"Oops, I guess I missed that. What did you get on the 11th and 12th holes?"

It didn't matter. Golf was our thing. I learned not to care about scores or hurrying up or losing my ball in the water or hitting out of a sand trap. I was happy to be swinging with John.

John kept playing golf. His last game was on July 21, 2023. He played with Tom, his best golfing buddy.

"How was your game, John?" I asked.

"I broke 100. I'm going out in style. I am going to pay for it tomorrow, but it was worth it. It was worth it."

John was changing again. It seemed like he'd lose some capability and then that would be a new plateau which became his home for a while. In 2022 involuntary movements, known as myoclonus, took over his body. It started with a small hand tremor in 2021. His neurologist tried to capture the tremors on video, but, of course, he did not shake in the doctor's office. The water does not drip when the plumber comes. It did not seem to be a big deal. One of his hands shook mildly, but it did not incapacitate him at all.

As time passed, both hands started shaking. Then it moved to his body. The shaking in his belly or chest impaired his ability to breathe,

2022: A Turning Point

We played golf together throughout our marriage. We had so much fun trying out different courses whenever we went on a trip somewhere, and we played on home courses many weekends either with friends or just the two of us. It was a social thing. Playing with John was like taking a beautiful walk in the park with your best friend. About the 15th hole I started to think about where we might have dinner and a nice glass of wine. We were both hackers, but John was a better hacker than me. John had a keen eye for the technical side of golf.

"John, help me. I keep hitting the top of the ball. I don't know why."

"Take a practice swing and let me see. Oh, you're too far from the ball, Erica. Just move closer—just an inch."

"Okay, let's see what happens." I swung and hit the ball a mile. "Thanks, honey. Next time you can tell me if you see something wrong."

He and I kept playing. Only close to the end it was different. He wanted to drive the cart and keep score as always. His memory lapses made it hard for him to keep track.

"John, go back. You passed my ball way back."

"Oh, sorry. I forgot about your ball."

"John, slow down. I am going to fall out of the cart. Did you put our scores down? I don't see anything for the last two holes."

"Oops, I guess I missed that. What did you get on the 11th and 12th holes?"

It didn't matter. Golf was our thing. I learned not to care about scores or hurrying up or losing my ball in the water or hitting out of a sand trap. I was happy to be swinging with John.

John kept playing golf. His last game was on July 21, 2023. He played with Tom, his best golfing buddy.

"How was your game, John?" I asked.

"I broke 100. I'm going out in style. I am going to pay for it tomorrow, but it was worth it. It was worth it."

John was changing again. It seemed like he'd lose some capability and then that would be a new plateau which became his home for a while. In 2022 involuntary movements, known as myoclonus, took over his body. It started with a small hand tremor in 2021. His neurologist tried to capture the tremors on video, but, of course, he did not shake in the doctor's office. The water does not drip when the plumber comes. It did not seem to be a big deal. One of his hands shook mildly, but it did not incapacitate him at all.

As time passed, both hands started shaking. Then it moved to his body. The shaking in his belly or chest impaired his ability to breathe, so John was uncomfortable all the time. He had to struggle to get air into his lungs and I could hear him breathing as he walked down the hallway. I joked with him and told him, "I feel like I'm living with Darth Vader." He could no longer surprise me by sneaking up behind me to put his arms around me or steal a kiss.

The myoclonus not only caused breathing issues, but it also exhausted him. He started sleeping several hours a day. Many days in a row after John's coffee in the morning and after he finished reading the sports page and doing the crossword puzzle and Sudoku game, he said to me, "I'm having a bad day. I need to rest for a bit." He went into the TV room, sat in the recliner and sometimes turned on the TV and sometimes not, and then went to sleep. Many days he slept for two to three hours.

The neurologist recommended a myriad of tests to determine the cause of the myoclonus. All the test results were normal, so by process of elimination the physician determined the myoclonus was a symptom of Alzheimer's. It is not a common symptom, but it could not be attributed to anything else. The neurologist prescribed a drug that is used for seizures to stop the shaking. Of course, there are side effects to all drugs, but his reaction was violent. He became very angry with me.

"Erica, let me explain to you how a bullet goes through a body and kills a person."

"Geez, John. I don't really want to know. Can we talk about something else?"

"It's really interesting. Let me explain. A bullet's damage is related to how fast it goes through the body."

"Please, John, I don't want to hear this right now."

He screamed at me, "Well, damn it, Erica. I want to talk about it now and you need to listen to me! This is my house too and I can talk about what I want to talk about."

John was never a violent person. So, the drug was stopped before we even knew if it could stop the myoclonus.

I wrote this on May 5, 2022:

The incidents of forgetfulness are now the norm. I know that whatever just happened is gone in a few minutes. I know that whatever is said lives for a moment in his brain. He is becoming detached, unengaged and listless. He sleeps for hours in an afternoon and it is difficult to get him up in the morning. Where did he go? It is so subtle that I don't realize how fast he is leaving me. Friends still think he is just fine."

One day John is my playmate and then, all of a sudden he is unable to gather the energy to go for a walk. I really can't understand this insanity—how am I supposed to watch the love of my life, my very best friend, my partner in everything, just slowly dissolve? How is he supposed to accept it?

John has spoken seriously of wanting to end his life before it is too late—before he is unable to do it himself. It is surreal that we have these conversations and I fluctuate between not believing this is happening and trying to imagine helping him die. Our lives have traveled from the sublime to total absurdity.

I try to relish our memories. We were (are) so in love and so happy together and totally hungry for each other. He held nothing back—this big, handsome, exuberant joyful man whom I have loved and loved."

In the Prologue I explain how I found the book, *In Love*, but I want to tell you how it affected both John and me and how it became part of our lives.

Many people are confused about right–to-die issues. This is one reason I wrote this book. California and Oregon and about twenty other states have laws that allow people to legally end their lives when they are terminally ill. California's law states that two doctors must swear an oath that the patient will die within the next six months and the patient must be mentally competent to make the decision on his own. These are the laws for committing a suicide with the help of a doctor.

However, this law negates the ability for someone with dementia to take advantage of it. First of all, no doctor knows how long a dementia patient will live. In addition, if a dementia patient who is otherwise healthy waits until he has only six months to live, he no doubt will be so far down the path of the progressive disease that he no longer has the mental capacity to make any decisions on his own.

It is a Catch-22. This makes it impossible for dementia patients to request the help of a doctor to end one's life on his own terms in the U.S. This is why *In Love* opened us up to explore our choices.

The book sent me reeling. I was in a pretty dark place after reading it. I felt confused and stuck. It was the beginning of getting what I, we, wanted but not wanting it. Now I needed to change my thinking from helping John live with a beastly degenerative disease to helping him die. *How can I do this?*

The most difficult issue I had was knowing that now I had to accept that a) there was a "way out for John" and b) I had to learn to accept John's fate. It seemed easier to handle John's illness like everyone else did—letting "nature take its course." Thinking, *Well, there isn't anything I can do about this. It was less stressful than knowing we could take action.*

Now I knew there was an alternative to suffering to the end of Alzheimer's, but if John wanted that option that would mean a premature death. I could not tell him about the book.

When I read it, John was having about four pretty good days in a row. He was shaking less and was more energetic, so I felt less threatened. I knew I had to discuss the Swiss option with him. I kept thinking to myself, *When is the right time to talk to John?*

I didn't want to approach him when he was doing so well. I didn't want to ruin his day or mine. When he was having a bad day, I couldn't discuss the book with him, because it just was not appropriate for several reasons: a) he wouldn't be able to comprehend the enormity of what we would discuss, b) he wouldn't remember anything we discussed, and c) I didn't want to add stress to an already difficult day.

I just carried it all with me. My life had changed to a life that was centered around John's disease and I felt a constant sadness in my brain and body. I saw no light at the end of the tunnel.

Our lives were polluted by the poison of John's disease.

After a few days, John started shaking again. I was simply in despair. I thought this was how I would spend the rest of my life—in a very sad place. I need to say this: *I am a happy person. This is just not who I am.*

I thought if I cried, then John would feel responsible, which would make me feel guilty about crying. I tried so hard not to cry in front of him, because I knew it would only make him feel bad and he did not need me to contribute to his anguish. But the situation made it tough for me.

I needed to speak to John about the book. We had to discuss his options to see what he would choose. I had been avoiding the issue for three weeks. I just couldn't find the right time and I suppose I didn't want to face what was probably going to happen.

On May 12, 2022, I wrote in my journal:

I have not spoken to any friends in a while and I don't feel like it. I like my little cocoon. Perhaps, I can just stay in it and be with myself. I'm the only one who understands what I feel, so I am comfortable with myself alone. People just feel like intruders into my world. Just John and me—this is what I want now.

Finally, around the middle of May, several weeks later, I got up the courage to have the discussion. At this point, there was no way John could read the book for himself.

He gave up reading at least a year ago. It is really hard to read when you can't remember what happened two pages ago. I gave him short books. I gave him books I knew he liked in his recent past. He started them and then I saw them left on the table untouched for long periods of time. When I finally asked him why he wasn't reading anymore, he explained to me his difficulty. So many signs of decline that each shot a pain through my heart.

I had to describe to him what *In Love* was about. I did the best I could explaining who Amy Bloom was and the process she went through to find Dignitas. I explained Dignitas' process and the requirements. I tried to give John a book report with as little emotion as possible.

When I finished talking, John asked me a few questions about the process and then told me he was certain he did not want to outlive his quality of life.

John: "Why do I have to travel to Switzerland? Tell me, again."

Erica: "Because there is no place in the US where you can do it legally."

John: "How does it work? How do I die?"

Erica: "They give you a drug so you don't throw up the real drug. Then, after that takes effect, they give you the lethal dose of some drug that makes you die. They say you fall asleep in minutes and then you die painlessly. You have to drink it yourself. No one can help you."

John: "Okay. I get it. I guess this is what I've been hoping for."

It was on that day he decided, and I consented to start applying to Dignitas in August. I think we wanted to wait until summer fun was over.

Our conversation was very strange. It is a very weird conversation to have with someone you love so much, but somehow, I stayed sad place. I need to say this: *I am a happy person. This is just not who I am.*

I thought if I cried, then John would feel responsible, which would make me feel guilty about crying. I tried so hard not to cry in front of him, because I knew it would only make him feel bad and he did not need me to contribute to his anguish. But the situation made it tough for me.

I needed to speak to John about the book. We had to discuss his options to see what he would choose. I had been avoiding the issue for three weeks. I just couldn't find the right time and I suppose I didn't want to face what was probably going to happen.

On May 12, 2022, I wrote in my journal:

I have not spoken to any friends in a while and I don't feel like it. I like my little cocoon. Perhaps, I can just stay in it and be with myself. I'm the only one who understands what I feel, so I am comfortable with myself alone. People just feel like intruders into my world. Just John and me—this is what I want now.

Finally, around the middle of May, several weeks later, I got up the courage to have the discussion. At this point, there was no way John could read the book for himself.

He gave up reading at least a year ago. It is really hard to read when you can't remember what happened two pages ago. I gave him short books. I gave him books I knew he liked in his recent past. He started them and then I saw them left on the table untouched for long periods of time. When I finally asked him why he wasn't reading anymore, he explained to me his difficulty. So many signs of decline that each shot a pain through my heart.

I had to describe to him what *In Love* was about. I did the best I could explaining who Amy Bloom was and the process she went through to find Dignitas. I explained Dignitas' process and the requirements. I tried to give John a book report with as little emotion as possible.

When I finished talking, John asked me a few questions about the process and then told me he was certain he did not want to outlive his quality of life.

John: "Why do I have to travel to Switzerland? Tell me, again."

Erica: "Because there is no place in the US where you can do it legally."

John: "How does it work? How do I die?"

Erica: "They give you a drug so you don't throw up the real drug. Then, after that takes effect, they give you the lethal dose of some drug that makes you die. They say you fall asleep in minutes and then you die painlessly. You have to drink it yourself. No one can help you."

John: "Okay. I get it. I guess this is what I've been hoping for."

It was on that day he decided, and I consented to start applying to Dignitas in August. I think we wanted to wait until summer fun was over.

Our conversation was very strange. It is a very weird conversation to have with someone you love so much, but somehow, I stayed disconnected. It is only because of this I could separate my being from all these conversations we had and would have that I could get through our talks.

In the days that followed John's decision to apply to Dignitas, his uncontrollable shaking became more persistent and violent. They exhausted him to the point where he slept most of the day.

One morning I asked him, "What would you like for breakfast?"

"I don't care."

I looked at his face and thought, *This is going to be one of those bad days. I feel so sorry for him.*

New symptoms started to show their ugly heads by the beginning of June 2022. John started making up stories. Delusions are a part of Alzheimer's, but at the time I thought he was making up stories because he couldn't remember what really happened, so he'd just fill in the holes. One night we were watching TV together, and we both had been quiet for some time.

All of a sudden, John broke the silence by accusing me, "Why are you ragging on me like this? You can't keep doing this, Erica." It was like one would imagine a schizophrenic behavior. Events like that scared me even though I knew it was the disease and not John.

There were other times when John asked, "Erica, why did you change the channel? I was watching that program."

"John, I didn't change the channel."

Without warning, the remote went flying past my face as he threw it as hard as he could.

John also would not eat unless I put food in front of him. I had to take over giving him his meds, because he could no longer remember to do it himself. His were not just memory changes. He was so drained of energy that much of what we did that was always fun for him now became difficult. We no longer rode bikes or walked to the Bridge. He started to play only fifteen holes of golf. He wanted me to decline dinner invitations and he gave up his theater tickets. "I'm sorry, Erica" became way too common in our home.

I did not correct John unless it was important. I did not want to embarrass him or make him feel bad. It was important to me to let John keep his dignity.

He began to perseverate. Tom asked John, "Can you help me work on the Napa house on Thursday?"

"Sure," John agreed on Sunday night. From that moment on John asked me repeatedly, "When am I supposed to help Tom work on the Napa house? When do I go with Tom to Napa? Is this the day I help Tom with the house?" Over and over and over again, he asked. It was a form of anxiety. It was another symptom I needed to become comfortable with.

Sometimes I felt annoyed and impatient with the repetition. I also felt like I would crack under the weight of all the newly added dysfunctions. But mostly I knew I had to keep myself together and calm to help John and me.

John no longer started conversations with me, nor could he engage in a conceptual conversation. Losing John's companionship not only made me feel lonely, but caused me to think,

This is what it will be like one day, only worse. I cannot imagine how much I will miss his presence. One of the terrible things about Alzheimer's is that regardless of where one is in the disease, one always knows it shall only get worse. There is no hope for the future. There is no thinking that maybe he will get better. The only direction is the one towards the end of life.

My heart broke over and over and over.

John reminded me, "Erica, you know you will need to be the one to decide when we go to Dignitas."

I felt crazy. John put a huge responsibility on my head. Who chooses when her husband shall die? Who does that? How do I do that? This certainly was not how I had expected our golden years to go. I could only hope I would have the wisdom and strength to do what he wanted.

The next set of decisions we had to make was who would we tell. The idea of informing one's loved ones and friends that you were planning your early death was completely unreal to me. First, I thought that we should not tell anyone until John was approved. It seemed reckless and inconsiderate to worry people about something this serious if you have no idea if it will actually happen. So, for a long time we said nothing. We held the possibility of Dignitas in our own heads for several months.

In spite of all this or maybe because of it, we took our last big trip together in September.

A Promise Kept

We had a memorable time traveling through the Bordeaux region of France for two weeks and one week in Paris. Alzheimer's worries were put on hold.

At the same time, we were planning a trip to Egypt with friends in October of 2023.

We kept living our lives. We kept planning, but in the back of my mind was always the thought that I had no idea what our lives would be like. I did not know if John could actually travel to Egypt. Would he be healthy enough? I made sure I insured the trip thinking I could cancel at any time.

France was both a wonderfully fun and memorable trip for us, but at the same time it was difficult. Fortunately, I planned the trip to allow flexibility in our schedule. John needed to nap each day and we had the space in our plans to allow for his needed rest. I did all the driving, planning, deciding, and navigating.

John was always in good humor and happy to be vacationing with me. We drank a lot of red wine and ate a whole lot of delicious cheese. I shall always remember how much he loved Paris.

I had wanted to go to Paris with John because he had never been there. I wanted to celebrate our wedding anniversary in Paris with John—April in Paris, but the weather is lousy in April so we waited until September. John could not have been any more enthusiastic about the beauty, elegance, and architectural feats of Paris. He absolutely loved the Eiffel Tower. I am so grateful we had the opportunity to enjoy Paris and the wine country together. Another memory for me. I'll always have Paris.

September 23, 2022

France

I know for sure now this is our last big trip. John just doesn't have the stamina. I feel so sad that he feels unwell and then he feels bad for me that he lacks the energy to do the things we used to do. He was completely different last year in Spain. He traveled relatively well last year.

This year in France he needs to sleep for a few hours in the afternoon and he never feels good—never feels like he has energy. He doesn't remember events from a day ago nor an hour ago. He has no sense of direction. He lacks the ability to engage with me and with what we see and do. He hardly spoke to our guide yesterday which is odd because John always loved to talk to our guides—actually he even likes to talk to the Uber driver.

I write this as a record, not a complaint. I'm really concerned about the near-term future. I can't help feeling hopeless. I miss my playmate so much.

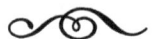

And So It Goes

Babies crying
Sleep comes
Oceans roar
Tides change
Anger flares
Peace reigns
Music blasts
Notes rest
Life screams
Death silences.

Breakfast Talk

Dan and I sat at a table in a breakfast diner somewhere in Palatine, Illinois where he and his family live. I liked stealing him away from everyone when I got a chance. I didn't often have the opportunity to get his full attention, so I looked forward to these moments. I ordered Eggs Benedict and he asked for salad with chicken on it. His usual. I had coffee; he had water.

I wanted to update him. "Dan, John is not doing well. His memory is getting really bad, and he is starting to decline in other ways. The shaking is making him very tired."

Dan answered, "Ya Mom, I see him sleeping a lot. I am sorry you both have to go through this." Dan paused to think for a moment. Then, he plunged right in. "Have you thought about suicide for John?"

He took my breath away. Where did that come from? I knew that someday soon John and I would need to tell our kids about what we decided, but I never expected anyone to suggest suicide.

I worried how and when we would tell them. I worried about how upset they would be. I worried if they would understand or try to dissuade us.

This was not a question I expected from any one of them.

I looked at the yellow of the eggs running on my plate and wondered *how do I talk to my son about this*? I was entering a strange world leaving my cocoon of secrecy. Danny waited patiently. After a few minutes, after I gathered my composure, I said, "Strange that you should suggest that. We actually have a plan. We were not ready to tell you kids yet, but since you brought it up, I'll explain it to you.

"John just doesn't want to live to the end of his disease. It gets pretty awful and he doesn't want to suffer through it. Besides, John is adamant that his brain is who he is and he doesn't see the point of living when he no longer is himself."

Dan is a quiet and thoughtful person. He listened to me without asking questions and then he asked, "What are you going to do, Mom?"

I paused and thought to myself, *How do I dive into this with my son*? I began to explain. I told him about In Love in as much and as little detail as I needed.

Dan asked, "Why do you have to go to Switzerland?"

"Well, because it is illegal everywhere else," I explained.

Dan pushed further, "But I thought it is legal in California."

"Ya," I said, "that is what most people think. It is only legal if you get two doctors to swear an oath that you will die within six months AND you have to be mentally competent to make the decision on your own. Dementia doesn't fit that law."

"Why not?"

"Because doctors don't know when a dementia patient will die. John could live with this for ten years. He is totally healthy otherwise. And by the time he is within six months of death, his brain will be long gone. He won't be able to prove he can make a decision on his own. He can barely do that now."

I held my head in my hands for a few minutes and then sipped my coffee, waiting for his response.

Dan sat quietly, looking at me. I had no idea what he was thinking. John was his best friend, his stepfather who taught him to drive, took him to school when he was a kid, who helped him fish, tutored him in math and made him laugh. I begged him, "Please don't tell anyone else. We are not ready for the family to know. Of course, you can tell Gretchen, but no one else."

He promised his silence. "When are you going to do this?"

"I am not sure, honey. It is a complicated process. We just started working on all the documentation. We don't even know if he will be accepted. We need to do it before John can no longer pass the mental capacity exams. We are trying to push it out as far as possible, but not miss our window of opportunity. We are threading a needle."

"I'll go with you, Mom. You can't do this alone."

It was then I had to hold back my tears. Finally, I said, "Thank you, Danny. But please think about what you are volunteering to do. It will be a very difficult time."

"I know," he said. "I will go with you."

The Popcorn Kernel

The kernel of popcorn stuck in his teeth. The small, white, buttery piece brought him so much pleasure. Sometimes he tossed a few M&Ms or Junior Mints in with the kernels of corn. He was not choosy.

Movies were our best date nights, spontaneous and random. There are two theaters on Chestnut Street just a few blocks from our house. On a night when we had nothing planned—and there were no Warriors games—I'd suggest, "Wanna go to a movie tonight?"

"What's playing?" John would ask.

"I'll check my app. There's a new Marvel movie at the Presidio at seven o'clock. It's supposed to be a good one. Owen said he liked it."

We held hands as we walked up to Chestnut. When it was chilly, John put my right hand into his left jacket coat pocket and put his hand in too to keep mine warm.

Most of the time we skipped dinner to have empty stomachs and no guilt to eat our popcorn with delight. John ordered the large with butter while I ordered the small with butter in the middle and the top. Usually, we got a large Diet Coke that we shared even though he preferred regular Coke. John started eating his popcorn eagerly as soon as he sat in his seat. He dove in with his strong hands and pulled out a fistful of the fluffy white kernels and stuffed it into his mouth. I, on the other hand, cannot touch my popcorn until the director's name is on the screen. John understood my rules, because I have stuck to this small bit of peculiarity ever since I can remember. We did not share our popcorn or there would be none for me by the time the movie started.

Fortunately, we enjoyed the same kind of movies. Neither of us could tolerate horror films and usually opted not to see foreign films with subtitles although we'd see one if it had really good reviews. Action movies that were just a lot of action and not much story were not our favorites, but Mission Impossible movies were good for an entertaining night.

Irish movies were always a problem. They were always sad, and we knew it. We went and then at the end we'd say to each other, "It was an Irish movie."

The best movies were any kind of movie with a good story. We both loved good stories and good acting. John had no problem seeing 'chick flicks' with me. I remember counting the number of men who slipped into the theater when we saw The Sisterhood of the Traveling Pants. I think John was one of five or six. The thing is he liked that movie. It had a good story. And his male ego was never an issue.

John hated movies with no endings. The problem is you don't know what's going to happen until the end of the movie. I always knew what he'd do. He'd stand up at the end and give me a disgusted look. He'd say, "God, I hate it when they don't give me an ending.

The Popcorn Kernel

The kernel of popcorn stuck in his teeth. The small, white, buttery piece brought him so much pleasure. Sometimes he tossed a few M&Ms or Junior Mints in with the kernels of corn. He was not choosy.

Movies were our best date nights, spontaneous and random. There are two theaters on Chestnut Street just a few blocks from our house. On a night when we had nothing planned—and there were no Warriors games—I'd suggest, "Wanna go to a movie tonight?"

"What's playing?" John would ask.

"I'll check my app. There's a new Marvel movie at the Presidio at seven o'clock. It's supposed to be a good one. Owen said he liked it."

We held hands as we walked up to Chestnut. When it was chilly, John put my right hand into his left jacket coat pocket and put his hand in too to keep mine warm.

Most of the time we skipped dinner to have empty stomachs and no guilt to eat our popcorn with delight. John ordered the large with butter while I ordered the small with butter in the middle and the top. Usually, we got a large Diet Coke that we shared even though he preferred regular Coke. John started eating his popcorn eagerly as soon as he sat in his seat. He dove in with his strong hands and pulled out a fistful of the fluffy white kernels and stuffed it into his mouth. I, on the other hand, cannot touch my popcorn until the director's name is on the screen. John understood my rules, because I have stuck to this small bit of peculiarity ever since I can remember. We did not share our popcorn or there would be none for me by the time the movie started.

Fortunately, we enjoyed the same kind of movies. Neither of us could tolerate horror films and usually opted not to see foreign films with subtitles although we'd see one if it had really good reviews. Action movies that were just a lot of action and not much story were not our favorites, but Mission Impossible movies were good for an entertaining night.

Irish movies were always a problem. They were always sad, and we knew it. We went and then at the end we'd say to each other, "It was an Irish movie."

The best movies were any kind of movie with a good story. We both loved good stories and good acting. John had no problem seeing 'chick flicks' with me. I remember counting the number of men who slipped into the theater when we saw The Sisterhood of the Traveling Pants. I think John was one of five or six. The thing is he liked that movie. It had a good story. And his male ego was never an issue.

John hated movies with no endings. The problem is you don't know what's going to happen until the end of the movie. I always knew what he'd do. He'd stand up at the end and give me a disgusted look. He'd say, "God, I hate it when they don't give me an ending.

I watched for two hours waiting to find out what happened and then they didn't tell me. It was a waste of time and money."

I'd often agree with him, but sometimes I'd think, *Well, life is a movie with no obvious ending.*

Popcorn and movies were our thing. We went alone. We went together. They were part of our good story. We had our beginning and middle and now we were reaching The End.

Trains

I understood John's fascination with trains. We both liked trains, but where it was all about the experience for me, it was about the machine for John. He relished machinery—after all, he used to build machines. He especially loved a good old-fashioned steam engine. I think he even liked Thomas the Train, which we read to Owen religiously and watched the DVDs repeatedly.

Many years ago I surprised John for his birthday with train tickets from the East Bay to Reno.

We sat in our seats, which faced wide windows giving us an unencumbered view. John asked, "Okay, now you can tell me where we are going."

"Yup, we are headed to Reno."

"Oh, that is so great, Erica. I've always wanted to do something like this."

"Well, sit back and relax. This trip is going to take about seven hours."

"That's fine. Pretty soon we are going to leave the flat lands and start uphill. I bet it's going to be spectacular."

"Are you hungry now, John, or do you want to wait to get something to eat?"

"Let's wait a bit and then we can enjoy a glass of wine and have lunch while we watch out the window. This reminds me of the train ride we took from Boston to New York. Only the scenery is going to be so much nicer."

The train climbed the Sierras while we watched out the windows. We were definitely not disappointed nor bored. "This may have been the best birthday present ever," John said at the end of our celebration.

We rode trains in Europe, as many do, and they lived up to their reputation as on time and clean. We took our grandkids to Felton near Santa Cruz to ride the steam engine through the redwood forest and we often took the Muni train to the Warriors stadium. Muni is the best deal in public transportation when the Chase Center is a full house.

But John's favorite train is the freight train that runs through Truckee. We often stayed at the Truckee Hotel when we skied at Squaw Valley. The hotel provides earplugs for its guests to block out the sounds as it rumbles through town each night.

Truckee is an old-fashioned logging town on the Truckee River. It was on the Trans-Sierra wagon road in 1863 and became part of the Central Pacific Railroad in 1867. The train tracks still run through the middle of town and veer up the mountain to provide a lovely quaint scene. John fell in love with this train and town. When we stayed at the hotel, he never cared that we had to share a bathroom down the hall or be awakened by the train each night.

Twenty-five years ago, when we bought the building we were renting, John gained access to do what he wanted in the garage. He began his own journey. His dream was to build a small model HO scale train. John's two trains ran through a town he designed to look just like Truckee. His town was in a valley surrounded by the Sierras. It had a hotel, the train station, the Mexican restaurant, and one major street complete with shops and restaurants. Pine trees decorated the mountain sides and wildflowers bloomed by the sidewalk.

When I looked for John, I knew he was either working in the garden or in the garage building his train. He built the train on a platform on a pulley system. When he was not working on the train, he simply pulled the ropes, and the platform holding Truckee and the train rested above our car. When he wanted to work on the train, he moved the car backwards and let the pulley down.

The underside of the platform is filled with John's ingenious giant integrated circuit board. I used to ask him, "How is the train coming? Is it running?"

"Well, yes, it's running, but I need to change it. I want the two trains to pass each other before they go through the tunnel. I'll need to fix some switches."

"Oh, okay."

"How do you know how to do all this stuff? You are not an engineer."

"I don't know how I know. I just do it."

"Where did you get those tiny trees from?"

"Erica, that's amazing. One day I was riding my bike through the Presidio and I saw these plants. I realized a small branch off the plant looked just like a tree that grows in the mountains. I picked these plants. Isn't that cool! Do you think the town looks like Truckee?"

"Honey, it's perfect. I love the train station and the hotel looks just like the Truckee Hotel. I can't wait to see it all finished."

He worked for hours at a time. In the winter, when it was cold in the garage, he put a heater by his side. In the spring, he found an old radio so he could listen to the Giants game. In the summer, he kept the garage door open to let the fresh air in.

Our tenant's children were fascinated by John's train and by watching him work. John let all three push the buttons to make the train go faster and slower, forward and backward. Our friends often asked to see the train. They wanted to see the progress and admired John's creativity and technical genius. Everyone loved the storage system.

As his illness worsened, he worked less and less. Gradually, he stopped completely. He couldn't think through the complex tasks of building his train that were once so easy for him.

The unadorned train town and its tracks still rest above my car. I have given many train cars to family and friends as mementos of John. My train cars sit on the fireplace mantel as a memory for me.

John never finished his train. He never had any intention of finishing it. He told me, "Erica, it's not meant to be done. It's just supposed to be my ever-changing dream."

Erica Baccus

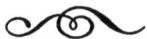

Freedom

Laughing, loving was he
Lonely am I
Losing himself into all he'd do
Loving him took my heart and brain
Last one to stop playing, he went on
Long ago I learned this is him
Let him go I think
Let me go he willed
Lovingly we embraced.

Anniversaries

We protect our marriage. We hold our love as though it were sacred. We celebrate each anniversary together on the day—not some day near it—but on April 17 and we do not invite anyone to join us in our celebration.

John was the one who started our surprise anniversary trips.

I pulled my car into our driveway on April 16—the day before our first anniversary. John was sitting on the front stoop waiting for me.

"Hi, Sweets. Give me a hug and go pack a suitcase, Erica. We are going on a trip."

"Really?"

"Yup, hurry up. I want to get on the road as soon as possible."

"What should I pack? Where are we going?"

"You have to guess where we are going. But pack casual clothes. Stuff for hiking and biking. Maybe one nice outfit for dinner."

"Awesome, this is so cool, honey. Are we going to celebrate our anniversary?"

"We are definitely celebrating."

I jumped into the SUV and saw a bottle of champagne and a dozen white roses. "Okay, let's play Twenty Questions, so I can guess where we're going. You have to tell me if I don't get it."

"Okay, go for it. I'm ready."

"Are we going somewhere north?"

"Nope. That is one."

"Have we been at this place before?"

"John chuckled, "Yup."

And so, it went until I guessed.

He took us to our favorite backpacking destination, Yosemite. Only this time we were going to sleep in a bed and eat gourmet food. We had reservations at the Ahwahnee Hotel in Yosemite. We hiked the valley floor and climbed Glacier Point, rode bikes all over, sunned ourselves by Mirror Lake, photographed wildflowers and stood in awe of Half Dome. I had no idea he had any plans to celebrate our first year together. It had to be one of the loveliest surprises of my life.

When our second anniversary neared, I thought, *John surprised me last year. I will surprise him this year.* I planned a weekend in San Francisco. As we were living in San Jose and didn't have a lot of leisure money to spend, San Francisco was a luxury for us. I found a quaint place called The Bed and Breakfast Inn on Union Street for our romantic getaway. I could see the Golden Gate Bridge from the bathtub. We had dinner at a fancy restaurant on April 17. The rest of the weekend we played tourists because we *were* tourists. John was delightfully surprised.

This second anniversary launched us into thirty-nine more surprise anniversary trips. John had the odd years and I the evens. We took our turns planning, while the other one guessed where we were going. One time we were at the airport and I still didn't know where we were headed. All I knew was what kind of clothes to pack and how long we would be away. As we got older and had bigger budgets, our trips became more lavish and adventurous. But, it didn't matter. What mattered was we spent a few days each year honoring our marriage and our love. Even in the years John had no idea where we were going, he found a way to get a dozen white roses into our hotel room.

I have a list of all forty-one anniversaries and where we went each year. They range from rafting down the Grand Canyon (John's trip) to golfing at the Boulders Resort in Carefree, AZ (my trip) to taking our first trip to Africa (my trip) to beaching it in Tulum, Mexico and visiting the ruins (John's trip). On our 26th year—my year to plan—I had to have hip replacement surgery.

"John, Dr. Calendar wants to schedule my hip replacement for April 17. What do you think of that?"

"Well, you should go ahead and do it. You are in a lot of pain."

"Yes, but it is our anniversary. We always honor our anniversary."

"Erica, sometimes life gets in the way. We will just postpone our anniversary. It is your turn this year and I will hold you to it. I am not letting you off the hook."

"Okay. I guess you are right. I know I will feel so much better once this is done. I'll have a brand-new hip."

So, in July, I held up my end of our tradition and took us to Seattle for a long weekend where we ate ourselves silly at all the wonderful farm to table restaurants and Pike Place Market, explored the city, went to the top of the Space Needle, and just enjoyed ourselves.

During the COVID year, when we could not travel anywhere, I cooked a gourmet dinner for the two of us. I set our dining room table with our beautiful gold-and black-trimmed Wedgewood china, sterling silver, linen napkins and candles. Setting a colorful, elegant table has always been a creative endeavor for me. I take my time and try to create a special ambience for every occasion. It was an even-numbered anniversary, our thirty-eighth, so it was my turn to plan, but as usual I was the one surprised as the doorbell rang, and I received a dozen white roses just as I did each and every year. I carefully placed them on the table between the lighted candles.

I printed out copies of a list of all of our anniversary trips. I told John, "Okay, honey, you choose your top five and bottom five trips and I'll do the same."

During our dinner and long into the evening, we compared our selections—some the same; some not and we talked about each of our choices. We spent the whole evening reminiscing about our trips. We laughed so hard at some of them. We remembered them all- the best and the ones that were least best—and the evening turned out to be so very memorable.

"Ahwanee has to rank up there. It was our first," I remembered.

"Yes, I agree. We had a great time. I always remember our view from the window. We could see Half Dome. I thought that was pretty spectacular. I also put The Benbow up pretty high and, of course we have to include Africa as a top one."

"Oh my gosh, John. Do you remember the picture of me balancing on one foot on the redwood log in the rain drinking wine straight out of the bottle in the forest behind the Benbow? We had so much fun there. And that little golf course we played on the hill? Africa is in a category of its own, though."

"Erica, I think one of the least best was that weird B&B we stayed in at the Gold Country. I think it was Sutter Creek. But we laughed so hard. We turned lemon into lemonade. And then the next morning we tried to play golf, but the fog was so thick we couldn't see our balls in front of us."

"Ya, John. That is the anniversary I danced on the piano. Everyone was singing lyrics to songs and somehow I wound up on the piano."

"Gosh, Erica. There are so many wonderful memories here. I am so glad you kept a list. It all just floods back."

"I'm so grateful you started this tradition, John. It is my favorite thing we do. Next year it will be your turn and hopefully COVID will be over."

Those anniversary trips became the highlight of our year—each year. We both cherished planning them, being surprised by them and just enjoying our special time together honoring our commitment.

A Promise Kept

I still have so many of the anniversary cards John gave me and many he bought to give me for future anniversaries.

When January comes around, I look forward to what the year will bring. I think about my birthday, which is on January 29, and then I think about our annual ski trip with the grandkids the last week of March and then I think about our anniversary on April 17. It is simply my favorite day of the year and I look forward to it each year with joy and love in my heart.

Our last anniversary, our forty-first, was John's year to plan, but he could no longer handle that kind of major task. He could no longer manage details of arranging an event or even choose what clothes to pack. We planned it together. We wanted something simple, not too far away. Just a pretty place for us to be together and celebrate our life together. I found a sweet B&B in Ojai, California. It was a quiet place with comfortable rooms, a pretty garden and walking distance to most everything. We drove there from San Francisco.

We spent one night in Santa Barbara where we walked along the ocean, enjoyed a glass of wine on the pier, had a great seafood dinner and went to sleep early. The next morning, we left early to get to Ojai in time for our tee time. It was a gorgeous public course, and we had a really nice time playing. I am not a great player by any stretch of the imagination, but I enjoy the walk in the park and the occasional brilliant hits. John was a decent golfer and he had a really nice long ball and often he was a crazy good putter.

On our second day in Ojai, we decided to hike. The wildflowers were in bloom and the mountain we hiked offered us exquisite views of the valley.

Then at one point John said to me, "Erica, we have been here before. I remember this hike."

I told John, "Honey, this is a new hike. We have never been here before."

John pushed, "But Erica, I remember that house over there and this trail. I just know we have hiked here before."

That evening, the Warriors were playing in the playoff games so we searched for a bar where we could watch. This happened to us often on our anniversary trips since the Warriors have been NBA champs four times in the last ten years and we were devout fans. It has always been an adventure to find a place that would show the game—especially if we were out of state or country. One time in Mexico, an outside restaurant whose floor was sand and where no doors existed had a big screen set up in its bar area.

"Hola senor," John tried. I see you have a screen. Can you show American TV here?"

"Si, senor. What are you looking for?"

"My wife and I are big basketball fans, and our team is playing in the playoffs tonight. Is there any chance you could show it here?"

"Oh, yes. We can do that for you. Just tell me what time and I will do that for you."

John and I were the only two people in the restaurant who cared about the Golden State Warriors, but we had a blast watching our winning team on our anniversary night drinking margaritas.

It was fun. This night we sat at the bar right smack in front of the TV and ate barbeque sandwiches. A stranger sat next to John, and I sat on the other side of John. John is the kind of guy who knows no strangers. He makes friends with everyone in the elevator. He is "that" guy. So, John and the "Guy" started a conversation which I could hear from where I sat.

The Guy: "I am so glad I found this bar."

John: "Yeah, we love this bar. We come here all the time."

To say I was stunned is a huge understatement. I thought, *What on earth is going on here?* I did not comment on their conversation, but I was worried.

The next morning, I took my shower and dressed in my golf clothes. We had a tee time at a different course. It was a perfect day. John slowly got out of bed and carefully prepared to get in the shower when he turned to me to say, "Erica, I don't think I can play golf today."

I tried to be comforting and said, "That's okay, honey. I can cancel our tee time."

I did not care that we could not get a refund. I suggested, "We can take a walk or relax in the garden. What would you like to do?"

John asked so sweetly, "Can we just go home? I want to go home."

I realized then that he was sicker than I had feared. I said, "Of course, let's pack our things and go."

We both quietly threw our clothes in our overnight bags, walked down the stairs and I told the manager, "I am sorry, but we are leaving today. Everything is fine with our room, but we need to go home."

A few days after our anniversary, John had a neurology appointment on Zoom. It was the usual "How are you doing, John?"

"I'm doing fine."

Then it was my turn to ask questions. I told the doctor about the hike and bar incidents while John listened, and I told her that John needed to leave a day early. "What does all this mean?"

She listened intently to my narrative and said, "John is changing stages. What you are describing with the hike and bar incidents are not just mistakes. These are examples of delusions. John, I believe you are now on the cusp of major neurodegenerative disease."

Anniversary Card I Gave John on April 17, 2022

My dear loving husband—what a journey we've been on. I shall never be able to thank you for filling my life with such joy and love for forty years. How lucky I am.

While our next chapter may not be what we anticipated, it is part of our story. We shall live it with dignity, with gratitude and with love.

We shall hold each other tight with care, with purpose and with the greatest affection.

I love our story. I love our life. I love our journey. And it's all because we love each other with honesty and authenticity.

John, you shall always be the love of my life. Thank you for these forty years.

Erica

Notes from my Journal: January 7, 2023

I find I am spending more and more of my time thinking about dying and death. As I was cooking soup today, I asked Alexa to play Shenandoah and Simple Gifts. Those were two of the songs Terry selected for his memorial service. Of course, it brought tears to my eyes and my heart. My loneliness for Terry felt overwhelming.

But also, I started thinking about all the deaths in my life. It is not surprising at my age that I have lost many of my loved ones except I lost my brothers and my parents years ago. This all, of course, led me back again to thinking about John.

Last night I went to see a concert with friends and left John at home. He didn't feel well enough to go. I became obsessed with the idea that John had either committed suicide or died of natural causes while I was listening to music. I envisioned him dead in his chair and how I'd react when I got home to find him. I kept imagining the scene over and over and just wanted to get home to make sure he was okay. In one vision, I was calm and called Trevor to come help me. In another vision, I broke down hysterically. In yet another, I just sat with John all night before I called anyone.

Death and dying are now constant friends. I feel the loss and mourn the death of my life with John. I am broken-hearted for John, who so willingly accepts his fate and is now getting closer and closer to wanting to end his suffering. What scares me is he won't be accepted to Dignitas and we have no Plan B.

It is not surprising that I feel isolated from my friends. I walk with death on my shoulder pretending to be the same as they are. It is painful and energy-consuming to pretend, so I'd rather be alone. I get angry that people who know me best can't tell that I am otherwise occupied. Yet, it is my secret. I am getting comfortable with the shadow that tells me to get ready for the big day.

I go to sleep each night spooned with John, appreciating that we can still touch each other. From the first time I lay with John, I loved the hair on his arms and it still comforts me today.

Measuring

I decided to start rating John's days. I believed it would be helpful to the doctors and to give John and me an accurate picture of what was happening in our lives. My scale resembled those I used in market research to get a subjective measurement. One translated to the worst day ever, 5 meant neutral and 10 signified a really good day. Sometimes I asked John to rate his day; sometimes I measured according to my perception. Below are my notes.

March 5, 2023:

John spent most the day sleeping. His Myoclonus tremors were so awful—so violent and debilitating. I was gone in the afternoon while he slept. He was so miserable physically. He told me, "I am being tortured, Erica. I don't want to live like this." He shook violently all the time he was awake.

Rating: 1

March 7, 2023:

John helped me hang artwork on our hallway walls. He was shaking mildly. He measured the photograph and the wall, but could not remember the measurements from the moment before. I started to write it all down quickly. We managed to get the job done. It took us about 1 ½ hours. Then he needed to rest. He slept for a while. He had a better day.

Rating: 4

March 8, 2023:

John went to his exercise class today. He took a shower and stayed awake. We are going to go to a movie tonight on Chestnut Street. This is a good day. Memory issues still apply but nothing out of the ordinary.

Rating: 6

March 9, 2023:

John did not do much. He said he felt low. He gave himself a rating of 3.

Rating: 3

March 10, 2023:

John helped clean a bit of the garage. He took a shower, and we went to the movies. He had a hard time walking to and from the theater. He was pretty alert.

Rating: 5.5

March 11, 2023

John had coffee in the morning and went back to sleep until 3P.M. He woke up at 10 a.m., so he slept from 11a.m.to 3 p.m. He didn't take a shower. He had no energy. He went back to bed for the night at 9:45 p.m. It was a day of sleep. I worry that this could be a trend.

Rating: 1

March 12, 2023

John showered and got out of bed around 9 a.m. He vacuumed the TV room. It is Oscar night and Vickie is coming over to watch with us. I think this gives him energy.

Rating: 7

March 15, 2023:

John had very bad shakes and very low energy today. He could barely talk. He asked me to cancel his exercise with Max. However, it was a nice day so he worked in the garden. I asked him, "How come you can work in the garden, but you can't exercise with Max?"

He explained, "I have to move very slowly and I can do that here in my garden. I can't exercise like that."

I can hear him breathe from the kitchen to our bedroom.

Rating: 2.5 (by John)

March 16, 2023:

John played golf today. He quit on the 15th hole because he was too exhausted to finish the game. He said he had trouble playing the first 15 because he was shaking and tired. He was really beat when he came home. This is the first time he could not finish 18 holes.

Rating: 3

March 17, 2023:

John sat in his chair all day shaking and tired. We had tickets to the theater and he bailed on me. He said he was shaking too much; he was too exhausted. He went down into the yard and said the climb up the thirty-two stairs was exhausting.

Rating: 2

March 18, 2023:

John had a really good day. He got up, showered, and worked in the yard. Caryn and Steve came over for dinner. John was like a normal person. He was the life of the party. He showed no symptoms of anything.

Rating: 7

March 20, 2023:

Another good day! It was sunny and nice outside. It took him until noon to get going, but then he worked in the garden again. Alex, Sylvia and baby Terry (named after his grandfather) visited us. John played with Terry and we had a nice dinner. Again, he seemed fine.

Rating: 6

Choosing The Date

How do I choose the date for my husband to die?

John had announced that this job needed to be my responsibility. He would not have the capacity to figure it out. We both knew his death would be premature given the circumstances. We both knew we wanted to wait as long as possible, but not miss our window of opportunity.

We were walking a tight rope. I was terrified that I would choose a date too soon and I was just as scared it would be too late.

We had no Plan B. I had to choose wisely.

Strangely, it turned out to be a matter of logistics. After the appointment with John's neurologist where his diagnosis had been advanced to John being "on the cusp of major neurodegenerative disease" I knew John's time was limited. It was time to move forward with plans. However, he had not yet been approved by Dignitas—he had not gotten his provisional green light. We had to wait.

Again, I thought, *I'm glad John has not been approved yet. I'm worried we could miss the opportunity.*

I waited each day checking my email.

There was a constant push-pull going on in my brain. Worried we would not get approved—worried we'd miss our window and anxious that it would all happen and much too soon.

Then, on May 10, 2023, I received this email from Dignitas:

Please be advised that a medical doctor cooperating with us considers an accompanied suicide to be justified in your case and thus has just given his consent to possibly write the prescription for you. However, the definite decision will only be taken after two personal consultations. You now have the "provisional green light" for an accompanied suicide in Switzerland.

I read the email over and over. *Did I understand what it said? I felt both relieved and frightened.* I felt sadness sweep over me in waves that couldn't wash away.

I needed to let John know that we were reaching the end.

"Oh, wow. Now what?" he asked. He seemed more interested in the logistics than the fact that he had just received approval to die. John's ability to think in the abstract was diminishing. Another insult to my heart.

I kept my promise. "Honey, I think it is time for us to set a date."

"Okay. Go ahead and do whatever you need to do. I trust you."

I began thinking about our lives. It was just May and we had summer plans. I knew for sure now we would not be going to Egypt in October. I had to cancel the trip. Owen was graduating high school on May 23 and his party was scheduled for June 4. It was important for John to be there—both for him and for Owen.

John needed to have another psychiatric exam and the report could not be more than three weeks from the assisted suicide. In addition, Dignitas required three to four weeks to prepare. This meant the date needed to be at least four weeks in the future.

I wanted time for John to visit our friends and give hugs one last time to his beloved family. I felt like we had the time for these goodbyes.

In the meantime, travel plans needed to be scheduled and Dignitas had a list of documents that I needed to complete to bring to Switzerland. I checked these documents over and over again to make sure I had them all and they were correct. I did not want to get to Zurich and have them tell me I am missing a document. I recall handing them the package and watching that no one looked at the documents I so carefully gathered. *Why aren't they checking them out?*

When I finally had it all straight it my mind, I sent a return email to Dignitas requesting the assisted suicide on July 26, 2023.

To Dignitas

John Baccus and I will arrive in Zurich on Monday, July 24. I understand John will have a doctor's appointment around 6:30 on July 25 in our hotel room and another one the morning of July 26. I have all the original documents with me and shall deliver them when we arrive. Please let me know if there is anything else I need to do or need to know.

Thank you for your help

A Promise Kept

Erica Baccus

While I had been tormented for months now on whether or not I chose too soon, John reassured me. In Switzerland the night before he died, he said, "Erica, we were so smart in choosing the right date."

I know I should have felt relief, but all I felt was fear.

"Provisional Green Light" May 10, 2023

Dear Mr. Baccus,

Please be advised that a medical doctor cooperating with us considers an accompanied suicide to be justified in your case and thus has just given his consent to possibly write the prescription for you. However, the definite decision will only be taken after two personal consultations. You now have the "provisional green light" for an accompanied suicide in Switzerland.

The following options are consequently available to you:

1. You accept the "provisional green light" as an emergency exit option to be made use of sometime later on, while you postpone the consultations with the doctor and the accompaniment until the time is right for you.

2. You contact us in order to arrange for only one consultation with the doctor, returning to your place of residence thereafter. You will decide on a second consultation with the doctor and the accompanied suicide later.

3. You contact us in order to meet the medical doctor two times within two or three days (depending on the doctor in question)

and to make use of the accompanied suicide, if the "green light" is confirmed, on one of the days thereafter.

By experience we know that the sole fact of having been given the "provisional green light" for an accompanied suicide might improve your condition, possibly rendering you able to further endure life and even to enjoy it to a certain extent. If you still have any questions, please do not hesitate to contact us.

In general, we need an approximate time frame of three to four weeks to accurately prepare the accompaniment of suicide. We kindly ask you to keep this in mind while planning your demise.

With the letter confirming that your request has been forwarded to one of the physicians collaborating with us, we already sent you the information leaflet regarding the necessary documents for the Swiss authorities. Once you wish to start the planning of your accompaniment, please send us these documents together with the enclosed papers, completed and signed ('AS Act', 'Data sheet for authorities', etc.). Please note the following explanations:

Power

According to the applicable provisions of Swiss Law, we are not authorized to directly obtain Sodium Pentobarbital (NAP). This is why we absolutely have to receive the aforesaid authorization form prior to the time of assisted voluntary-death proceedings at our office, so that we will be able to obtain on your behalf the medicament NAP from the pharmacy.

Since 1998, DIGNITAS has conducted more than 3,000 accompanied suicides which always led to the individual's chosen goal: a self-determined, safe and painless end of suffering and life. Whilst the individual wishing to have an accompanied suicide determines the time frame, two specifically trained team members will safeguard the correct practical and technical procedure so that everything adheres to Swiss law.

After taking the Sodium Pentobarbital—the medication used for accompanied suicides at DIGNITAS—the person will fall asleep within two to five minutes, slipping into a deep coma, a condition similar to general anesthesia. Only after a while of complete unconsciousness, the Sodium Pentobarbital affects the respiration which will become weaker and finally stops. In consequence, this leads to a natural dying phase. Usually, the time between falling asleep and dying lasts from 15 minutes to one hour. In very rare cases, due to a seldom anomaly of the stomach, the unconscious phase lasted several hours. In order to ensure that you achieve your goal even in such a rare situation, and that your dying phase is not disturbed by unauthorized third parties, we kindly ask you to date and sign the enclosed instruction and return it to DIGNITAS.

Please note that at the time of the assisted suicide an up-to-date report from the psychiatrist must be available which confirms beside your general conditions also your ability to judge and provides information about your orientation including cognitive abilities. The report must not be older than 2-3 weeks at the day of assisted suicide.

Yours sincerely

DIGNITAS

To live with dignity – To die with dignity

The Dentist

I arrived at the dentist's office just on time. I don't hate my dentist. He is drop-dead gorgeous, six–foot-something, broad shoulders, that perfectly symmetrical face and he is so very sweet. But I do hate going to his office for an appointment. I am not sure why. He has never actually hurt me. I just don't like anything about going to the dentist.

Today was especially difficult. I sat in the new office—decorated in contemporary mode—which is not my thing. It felt sterile—devoid of humanity. I tried to think about how to approach what I needed. I tried to not think of what I needed.

My appointment was with Desiree, who had been cleaning my teeth every six months for about thirty years. I rarely actually saw Dr. Franks because I had no need to actually see The Dentist. I didn't want to pay the extra money for him to look into my mouth and say, "Looks good to me. Good job, Erica. See you next time."

Dr. Franks had been my dentist for a very long time. John was also one of his patients. John was a reluctant patient. He fished around looking for the perfect dentist and finally succumbed to my "Please, just go to Dr. Franks. He will not suggest work on your teeth you don't need."

Every six months when I went to the front desk to pay my bill, Dr. Franks appeared out of nowhere, put his arm around me and asked, "How are you, Erica? How is John?" We talked about skiing and traveling around the world and his children and my grandchildren. We never talked about teeth.

Today was May 16, 2023. Desiree finished my cleaning. I asked her quietly, "Desiree, could I speak with Dr. Franks?"

"Sure, she said. "I'll go get him."

I waited nervously for him to get to our cubicle. He walked in, smiled hello and gave me a hug. Desiree left the area. "How are you, Erica? How is John?"

I said I was fine, but I needed to ask a favor. Without hesitating anymore, I asked Dr. Franks, "Do you have x-rays of John's whole mouth?" He very carefully and slowly answered, "Yes, I do. Why are you asking?" I could tell he probably had an inkling why I was asking, but he needed me to clarify.

He pulled up a stool and said, "Sit down, Erica." He sat opposite me looking at me squarely in my eyes. He leaned in as if to close the space between us, forearms on his knees, hands folded, "What's going on, Erica?"

As my eyes clouded over and my throat clogged, I knew I needed to confess the truth. John and I had not told anyone outside of our immediate family and now I had to tell this man. I was wary of his reaction. Would religious beliefs enter the conversation, would he just be a distant doctor doing what needed to be done, or would he understand? I so wanted him to be on our side.

I said, "John has Alzheimer's and has chosen to not live to the end of the disease. We are going to Switzerland in July. He will participate in an accompanied suicide there. The Swiss government requires an X-ray of his teeth."

I crossed my arms around my body literally holding myself together. Dr. Franks said, "I'm so sorry, Erica. I will get these for you right away. Just sit here for a few minutes."

Meanwhile, he started to tell me a story of his mother-in-law who had struggled through Alzheimer's to her end. He told me no one should have to go through this. He understood why John chose to end his life on his own terms. I had heard these stories before, but I needed reassurance that we were doing the right thing. I was relieved to know he had compassion for our decision. It was such a difficult decision that anytime someone expressed some kind of agreement I felt a tiny bit of comfort.

I walked out of the office with a folder full of pictures of John's teeth. Those teeth—all in a straight row which I saw every time he smiled at me. Those teeth he used to cut a piece of floss off or open a sealed package of salami. He had sharp teeth. Those teeth he used to nibble on my ear or cut a fishing line. The teeth he used to chew his steak and bite his beloved bread. The teeth that gave structure to his jawline. I loved his teeth as I loved every part of him.

Now those teeth would be used to identify his body.

Choosing My Escort

"I'll go with you, Mom." Those words from Dan would forever be in my brain. I knew it was important for me to choose the right person to help me get home from Switzerland. Amy Bloom spent some time explaining how and why she chose a friend. For a while, I thought that made sense: bring someone who would not be so devastated by John's death, but someone who cared about me and was cool and practical.

"I'll need someone I can trust to help with airplane stuff and get me on the plane without too much drama," I thought.

Then I thought, "No, I need someone who I can be comfortable with if I am a hysterical mess."

And while I was thinking all this, John was telling me, "Erica, I want Kyle and Lori to come to Switzerland."

I struggled with this decision. I believed John should have his children with him if that is what he wanted. I knew in my heart if it were me, I would've insisted Danny would be with me. I went round and round in my head on this, but I also wanted my last moments with John to be with me alone.

I knew that was selfish, but I kept picturing what it would be like with others around and that felt so inappropriate to me. I imagined myself in John's arms as he went to sleep—this was not a place for anyone else.

In addition, I believed none of the kids would do well actually watching John die. I knew it was going to be hard enough for me.

I had all kinds of arguments against this. "John, I understand you want your kids with you. But I don't want to worry about someone else's feelings when this happens."

"But I am the one who is dying and I want my family around me."

"Yes, it is you who will die, but it will be me alone afterwards."

"John, this is not like you are dying of cancer in a hospital and the whole family can come sit by your side and hold your hand. This is something else completely. Besides, you would not be doing Lori or Kyle a favor. This is going to be traumatic. No one wants to watch you kill yourself. I don't want to watch you."

Then I told John, "Honey, I feel like this is an intimate thing between you and me. I don't want anyone there at the time except me. It is about us."

We had this conversation over and over again. Like most conversations by this time.

Meanwhile, I was still figuring out who should help me get home. I went through all kinds of people in my thoughts. *I could ask Keith (Judy couldn't travel), or Anne, or Jennifer or Tom and on and on. I let it all sit in my gut as I imagined myself crawling on the floor in tears in the middle of an airport. Who would be okay with that?*

I finally realized that Danny was the only person I wanted and he already offered. *He is my son. Next to John, I am closest to him. I can cry with him, and he can cry with me.*

I called him and asked him again, *Are you sure you want to go to Switzerland?* Then I asked, "Can I come home with you instead of going back to California? I don't think I'll want to go home right away."

I explained again to John why I needed Danny and then explained the logistics. "John, honey, Danny is not going to be in the room with us. He will come to the Dignitas house with us, but when it's time, he'll go to another room. Then he can take me to the airport. I'm going to go home with Danny. I don't want to go back to San Francisco right away. I think I am going to need some time and I can be around the boys and the family."

Finally, John agreed with me, or he forgot all about it. I don't know which.

Of all the things I wished I had done differently, this was one I did right.

Owen's Graduation

John and I looked forward to celebrating Owen's high-school graduation with him and the rest of the family. His graduation was on May 23, 2023. Owen excelled in high school even though he struggled with learning disabilities since kindergarten. He had trouble recognizing letters and numbers, which made learning to read extremely difficult. He learned to read just fine, but needed more time than most to finish an assignment. Owen was excited to start his freshman year of college in August at Arizona State. John and I were proud of him, but mostly happy that he was happy.

By this time, all of our children knew about Dignitas. We had not told the grandchildren. We had agreed with their parents that this was a discussion they should have with the kids.

Dan and Gretchen had told Owen and Noah that Papa's Alzheimer's was getting worse and they didn't know what the future held in store. As weeks passed and more questions arose. Dan and Gretchen decided they just had to tell the boys the whole truth. Owen and Noah learned about Papa's imminent death shortly before we arrived for the graduation.

We had a day to spend with the kids before the graduation. I tried to keep it normal. I never knew what John was actually thinking.

Did he remember how few weeks he had left while he was with the boys? I believe his awareness went in and out. Sometimes he grabbed a hug from Owen and Noah and sometimes he just hung out like normal.

"Owen," I said, "put on your cap and gown for us and give us a fashion show."

"Yeah, Owen," Papa seconded. "I want to see how you look. This is so exciting."

"Nah, you'll see me when I get ready tomorrow tonight. Papa, you wanna take Phin (the family dog) for a walk with me?"

"Sure, let's go. I'll challenge you and Noah to a Ping-Pong game when we get back."

"How many points do I need to give you?" Owen asked.

"Ha ha, big shot. I can still whip your butt. Where is Noah?"

"Poor kid, he still has school. He'll be home by 3."

Graduation Day arrived and the house was happy.

"Owen, you look awesome," I said. "I love the dark green. Let's get everyone outside for picture taking. Noah, can you get your mom and dad and Phin and come on out?"

"Yup, Gma, I'll try."

"Okay, first let's get Owen and Papa. Then Owen and Papa and Noah. Look over at me and smile."

"Can we get Phin in the photo?" Owen asked.

"Always. He's the best-looking guy in the family. Okay, now let's get the whole family."

On our way to the graduation, I told John, "Honey, your first grandchild is graduating highschool. Are we really that old?"

John said, "I'm really proud of him. I just hope he remembers to enjoy this day."

The graduation ceremony was awesome. Five hundred kids all dressed in vibrant green had their names called out.

We waited with all the other families in the parking lot for our newly minted college freshman. Finally, Owen appeared and his dad grabbed him in a hug.

Then Papa said, "Come here, Owen. I need to hug you. You did great and I am so very happy for you. Remember, next year to say Yes to as much as possible. Grab your brass ring."

Spring had broken into the Midwest winter. Sunny and warm days had arrived. We were a typical family taking pictures of the graduates in cap and gown, except as the family photographer I focused on taking photos of John with each grandson and family member. I thought these were probably some of the last pictures of John with our family. There was no escaping the melancholy I felt.

We left for the Lake House in Indiana the next day where Gretchen's huge family congregates every Memorial Day weekend. It was our first trip there.

John jumped right in. "Hi, I'm John. I'm Gretchen's father-in-law. Wow, look at all these little kids. Come on gang—someone grab a football."

Gretchen said, "John, we are going on the boat. Are you ready for the lake?"

"What do I need?"

"Just your water shoes, swimsuit and sunscreen."

"We will bring the drinks and food."

"Gretchen, I'll help carry stuff. Just tell me where to go."

"Okay, just bring a cooler over to the pier."

"Come on, kids, jump on. You try to stay on this floaty thing, and I'll make it shake."

"Yikes, this is fun," one of the kids yelled.

John warned, "I can shake you guys up all day on this. You are going to fall in the water. Let me know if you get tired."

Unfortunately, Dan got COVID right after graduation and could not join in the fun. John lit up every room and every event with his famous laugh and partying mood. Only the immediate family knew the truth, so reality could be set aside for a few days of fun. When we were invited to return for next year's Memorial Day celebration, I thought, "It will only be me next year."

We returned to Dan and Gretchen's house about one week before

Owen's actual graduation party. Unsurprisingly, John got COVID when we returned to their home, so he had to quarantine in the bedroom. On occasion someone in the family found John walking around the house. "Erica, John's out of the bedroom."

I rounded him up. "John, honey, you have COVID and you have to stay in the bedroom."

"Oh, I do? I feel okay now."

"Yes, you are taking medicine to feel better and shorten your isolation. We want you to be able to come to Owen's party next week."

"Okay, I'll go back to the room."

"I'll come hang out with you for a while. We'll both wear masks."

John recuperated well and joined the party on June 4. A bittersweet time, for when goodbyes were given, it was the last hug for Gretchen, Owen and Noah, or so we thought.

The Farewell Tour

Jennifer and David

We didn't really understand that Owen's graduation was the beginning of a long good-bye for John. It was not planned; the tour grew organically.

We always visited Jennifer and David in their Oregon home in the spring or summer. Jennifer, John and I worked together in the late 1970s and have been best friends ever since.

They come here in December. We have been taking turns for almost two decades now.

We had been through all kinds of jobs together, earthquakes, a vacation to New Zealand, family dramas and weddings, the births of our grandchildren, weekend trips, the deaths of their parents and all the other milestones friends of over forty years share.

On this trip, in early June, we planned to meet them in Florence, OR just to go somewhere different. It is a small quaint ocean town with some beautiful hiking trails and a few good seafood restaurants. We shared an Airbnb.

We met around lunchtime so we found a barbecue restaurant on the main drag of the town where we sat outside at a picnic table. Big hugs all around and John said, "Great to see you, Davey." Jennifer hugged John and asked pointedly, "How are you doing? "How was your flight? Florence looks like a cool town, don't you think?"

"Flight was easy. Yes, I never heard of this place before, but it looks cute."

"How is Gunnar?" I asked. Their dog was like their child.

"Our Airbnb is right over there across the street. You can see it from here," Dave said. We can dump our bags after lunch and then go for a walk."

We walked lazily to our place, walked up the stairs and picked bedrooms. Jennifer and David took the one that looked quieter. We didn't care. Then we sat down in the living room to chat and figure out our plans for the next two days.

But first we needed to tell them.

Kyle and the Kids

Visiting our Kansas family was easier. Kyle already knew and Haley and Drew only understood Papa was sick. They lived in a rural town outside of Kansas City on a lake in a big house with a swimming pool, a water-skiing boat, and every water toy you can think of.

It is always hot there in June, so we spent our time playing in the pool, riding in the new water ski boat and enjoying summer playtime with the kids.

The Farewell Tour

Jennifer and David

We didn't really understand that Owen's graduation was the beginning of a long good-bye for John. It was not planned; the tour grew organically.

We always visited Jennifer and David in their Oregon home in the spring or summer. Jennifer, John and I worked together in the late 1970s and have been best friends ever since.

They come here in December. We have been taking turns for almost two decades now.

We had been through all kinds of jobs together, earthquakes, a vacation to New Zealand, family dramas and weddings, the births of our grandchildren, weekend trips, the deaths of their parents and all the other milestones friends of over forty years share.

On this trip, in early June, we planned to meet them in Florence, OR just to go somewhere different. It is a small quaint ocean town with some beautiful hiking trails and a few good seafood restaurants. We shared an Airbnb.

We met around lunchtime so we found a barbecue restaurant on the main drag of the town where we sat outside at a picnic table. Big hugs all around and John said, "Great to see you, Davey." Jennifer hugged John and asked pointedly, "How are you doing? "How was your flight? Florence looks like a cool town, don't you think?"

"Flight was easy. Yes, I never heard of this place before, but it looks cute."

"How is Gunnar?" I asked. Their dog was like their child.

"Our Airbnb is right over there across the street. You can see it from here," Dave said. We can dump our bags after lunch and then go for a walk."

We walked lazily to our place, walked up the stairs and picked bedrooms. Jennifer and David took the one that looked quieter. We didn't care. Then we sat down in the living room to chat and figure out our plans for the next two days.

But first we needed to tell them.

Kyle and the Kids

Visiting our Kansas family was easier. Kyle already knew and Haley and Drew only understood Papa was sick. They lived in a rural town outside of Kansas City on a lake in a big house with a swimming pool, a water-skiing boat, and every water toy you can think of.

It is always hot there in June, so we spent our time playing in the pool, riding in the new water ski boat and enjoying summer playtime with the kids.

John and Kyle gabbed about stuff like always:

John: "Kyle, are you going to do your light show for the fourth of July?"

Kyle: "Oh, ya. It's going to be better than ever. I'm inviting Drew's whole soccer team over and I'm going to choreograph the best fireworks.

John: "I wish I could see it."

Kyle: "I'll take some pics, Dad."

John: "Let's get the kids and play frisbee in the pool. Come on, Erica, jump in."

Kyle: I'll get the frisbee. Dad, you get Haley and Drew."

One may think this was an impossible situation, to play in the water while John and I were counting the days of his life he had left. I know Kyle showed his game face with his kids but had trapped his emotions inside of himself. His dad was visiting his grandchildren to say goodbye.

The Fourth of July

Next trip. Another annual tradition. John and I always spent the Fourth of July at Tom and Cheryl's house in Lake Tahoe. It was usually a long weekend of partying: golf, picnics, outdoor concerts, fireworks, hikes, and great dinners.

Our time with our Tahoe friends is mostly spent skiing or playing golf and sometimes traveling together. Intimacy happens on a one-on-one basis while group activities are kept sort of on the "let's have fun" basis. Strangely enough, two of our friends were in the midst of cancer treatments themselves during this holiday weekend and were doing quite well with their treatments. But it was a concern for all of us.

As I was packing for the trip the day before we left, John asked, "Do we have to go? I'm tired."

"John," I urged. "Honey, this is your last chance to see your friends. This is your only chance to say goodbye to them. Even though they won't know you are saying goodbye, you will."

John acquiesced and he had fun playing golf and goofing around with Brian, Tom, Mike, and Barry. We had agreed not to tell anyone about Switzerland. It was a party weekend and didn't seem appropriate to destroy everyone's fun. At one point, though, I watched John walking away with his arm around Brian and a beer in his hand. I wondered what he was saying. It really didn't matter anymore what he said or to whom.

On the morning of July 4, Cheryl and I were taking a ride into town. She needed something from the drugstore, so I went along to keep her company. John and Tom hung out at home together. They hung out well together.

Cheryl drove along the curvy mountain road. We were just chatting about nothing important and then she asked, "Erica, have you made up your mind about going with us to Egypt in October?"

I snapped, "Cheryl, John is going to be dead in twenty-two days, so no, we are not going to Egypt."

I turned my head to look at Cheryl as the tears slipped down her face and the car swerved towards the cliff. She pulled to a stop as soon as she could. I needed to explain.

Through her tears she begged, "John has to tell Tom. You can't tell me and not Tom. He is going to be devastated."

"I know. When we get back to the house, I'll tell John what happened and ask him to tell Tom."

The Surprise Visit

Kyle and Lori made plans to spend the last weekend with us at our home. It was their goodbye. However, one afternoon Noah called me to ask, "Grandma, Owen and I want to see Papa one more time. Can we come?"

"Oh, Noah, that is so wonderful. I just need to check with Lori and Kyle to make sure it is okay with them to share the weekend with you two."

Both Lori and Kyle were happy to have the boys join them. They actually thought Owen and Noah would lighten the atmosphere and help make the weekend a bit easier.

Lori, Kyle, Noah and Owen played poker with John. I heard lots of guy jokes and John won a bunch of money. We went for walks in the Presidio and sat in John's lovely garden. I tried to stay out of the way to let them have whatever conversations they needed to have. It turned out to be a joyful weekend bathed in love and laughter. I was so grateful to our two grandsons for their courage and love. I was so sad for each of them as they hugged John for the last time at the airport.

Each farewell tested my resilience, discipline and my energy. I had hosted all the farewells—all the last moments—and now in a few days it would be my time.

Erica Baccus

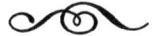

Hard Times

Why did you think I could do this
I cannot be without you
Why did you think I was strong enough
I never said I could
You should have asked me
You said I'd be okay
I cannot do this
It is just too hard—this stuff.

Traditions

Every family has its own traditions. They come about organically while some, like putting the star on top of the Christmas tree are handed down generation to generation or communicated through our culture.

Ours were important because they were part of what made us unique. They provided a glue for marriage and a map to tell you how you are supposed to live as a family.

I now have no one with whom to share our traditions. They are now empty dates and events that can't exist yet are filled with memories. I shall keep these memories in my heart because he and I created them together. Our traditions were born out of our desire to have fun with each other, love each other and give to each other.

Our anniversary trips, regardless of how big or small, or simple or extravagant, gave us each time to remember why we chose to be married. These trips offered us moments to reflect and sign up for another year of love. No matter where we were on April 17, we had a lovely dinner out where we could toast each other for our lives well spent. White roses magically appeared in our room saying, "Erica, I will always remember my gratitude for having you in my life." The roses were John's way of telling me how much he loved me. Pure and white and real.

As April 17 passed, I missed John from within the core of my body, but I also experienced gratitude for having had a marriage where we both understood the importance of our union. Gratitude occupies one part of my brain, while another part is consumed by the claws of grief. The truth is I wish John were still alive.

Putting up our Christmas tree became a tradition. Yes, many families make a big deal of it and we were no different. But we had our own things. In the early years, we cut down our own tree from a forest that offered us axes and a bag. We brought a bottle of wine and picnicked where we found a clearing. When we moved to San Francisco, we drove to the nearby junior high Christmas-tree parking lot to buy the biggest one we could fit in our living room. I loved these trips, because the sales guys were always from Australia or New Zealand with charming accents and strong bodies.

John always needed to trim the trunk himself when we returned from the lot to our garage. It had to be perfect. He and I dragged the tree into the living room and stood it up, trying so hard to get it straight. The best part was John built a self-watering system for the tree. He took a pail, wrapped it in Christmas wrapping paper, put a hose into the pail at one end and the other end in the tree. Then he filled the pail with water. The hose sucked up the water from the pail and delivered it to the tree. No one knew anything other than it looked like we had a big present under the tree, and we always had a freshly watered tree.

This was John. He fixed things even when I didn't know they needed fixing. If you couldn't buy the fix at the store, he imagined it and made it happen.

Most people have to water their trees. I didn't.

He trimmed the tree with the lights and we both hung the ornaments. Each was from a trip we took together or something one of our kids or grandkids made or some special nod to our favorite things, a camera for me, a greenhouse for John. It took a long time to hang all these memories because we talked about each one. The last one was a star Danny made in kindergarten out of paper that goes on top of the tree. One would think it would be destroyed after 50 years, but I have given it the care it deserves, and it survives.

When we moved back to San Francisco from Boston, I invited our San Jose friends to our home for a Christmas brunch. These were the soccer parents; parents of the boys Dan played soccer with when he was twelve. Although the boys are no longer close, somehow, we, the parents, maintained our own friendships. I wanted to make sure we could celebrate our friendship each year even though we lived fifty miles apart.

Each year I combed through brunch/breakfast cookbooks for a tantalizing recipe. Each year I served homemade cinnamon coffee cake, rum cake and my mother's recipe for eggnog, which is really not eggnog. It is made with Everclear alcohol, lots of eggs, powdered sugar, milk and heavy cream. I set the table with Christmas colors and decorations. It was always a lively, joyous, festive occasion and a chance for us to catch up with each other.

The doorbell rang. The door opened at exactly 11:00 AM and in walked Bev, Pauline and Bobbi. Les was parking the car and, in a few minutes, the rest would arrive.

"Merry Christmas, everyone," I called from the kitchen.

A Promise Kept

"Let me have your coats," John offered. "What would you like to drink? Coffee, mimosa, wine or Erica's eggnog? We have plain juice too."

"Oh, I want to start with that wonderful eggnog from Erica's mother's recipe. Nothing like it," claimed Bev.

"Okay, let's get the news on the boys and all the grandchildren." I always looked forward to finding out how all our soccer boys were doing.

"Wow, something smells really good. As usual. What's cooking, Erica?" Bill wanted to know.

"Well, there is the usual rum cake and cinnamon coffee cake and I have a new frittata in the oven. David is going to make the sausage."

And so, it went. Every year for twenty-nine years.

My first brunch was December 1993. There were sixteen at the table. My last brunch was December 2022. There were nine of us. Time has taken John and Les since then, so my brunches are completed. It was a lovely tradition that kept friendships alive and served us all with a continuing commitment to each other.

Lox and bagels on Warriors' game nights, popcorn at the movies, two turkeys, one roasted and one barbecued for Thanksgiving, making bacon with Owen and Noah and John's special recipe for French toast were all traditions we kept.

We nurtured our lives with food and intention and love.

Medical Mania

John was required to complete two psychiatric exams to demonstrate to Dignitas that he had the mental capacity to make the decision to die on his own—that he understood what he was preparing to do and that he was not influenced by anyone including me. It was one of the requirements that dictated how much longer he could live.

"We require a medical report of a **psychiatrist** confirming that you are an **autonomous personality** who, even in relation to life-essential decisions (1), is **capable of recognising your own situation** (capacity to understand) and of **drawing conclusions from this understanding** (capacity to appreciate) with of a view to putting into practice any insight gained and **decision taken without submitting to influence by third parties** (will power and decision-making power)."

The first exam was scheduled in early 2023. John and I again traveled to UCSF this time to meet with a psychiatrist. She interviewed John for about two hours and then asked me to corroborate certain facts afterward. At the end I asked, "Dr. Shrink, do you think you will give John an approval. Will he be able to move forward with this process?"

"Oh, yes, I don't see any problems. He is very clear about his decision. I can have the report finished within two weeks."

"Whew, that is a relief. Thank you very much. Then, I'll check MyChart for the report in two weeks?"

"Yes, I am sorry to meet you under these conditions. I wish you well."

Two weeks came and went. Four weeks slipped by. No report. I was getting anxious.

What is the problem? We are going to miss our deadline.

I emailed our social worker on our palliative care team. Geoff was my right-hand man who helped me navigate the oceans of documents and rules. He was a liaison with the neurologists, and other attending doctors. "Geoff, Dr. Shrink promised she'd have John's mental capacity report four weeks ago. I still don't have anything. Can you help me out here?"

"Oh, so sorry, Erica. I'll see what I can find out."

A few days later: "Erica, there is a problem with something a neurologist said about John. I will get it figured out for you."

Six weeks after the appointment I had a Zoom meeting with Geoff, the attending physician and John's current neurologist.

I asked, "Can someone tell me what is going on? Why don't we have the report? It wasn't supposed to be a problem."

Geoff explained, "Well, what I know so far is Dr. Shrink will not sign off on her report because somehow John's diagnosis in his medical chart is not the same as the one she has in her history. They have to match."

I have always been very polite with doctors, nurses, hospital staff and anyone who has anything to do with power over my health or my kid's or John's.

But I exploded. "WE DON'T HAVE TIME FOR YOUR MEDICAL BUREAUCRATIC BULLSHIT. THIS IS A LIFE AND DEATH SITUATION FOR JOHN AND WE NEED THIS FIXED NOW."

Then, of course, I apologized. Geoff consoled me with, "Erica, you do not need to apologize. I know what it means to advocate for someone you love. You were advocating and you have every right to be upset. We will get this fixed this week."

John's second mental capacity exam needed to be sent to Dignitas no more than three weeks before his *death date*. Thankfully, Dr. Shrink was out of the country on vacation—although she really wasn't the problem, I couldn't help hold her responsible. I needed to find another psychiatrist who could conduct the exam for us. Geoff recommended Dr. Booty. I called him.

Once I explained the situation, who referred me and what we needed, Dr. Booty made an appointment for us on Zoom for a date that would meet the three week requirement.

To my surprise both John and I were included in this appointment.

John was his usual sunny, cheerful self. I never knew if his disease was affecting his ability to understand the seriousness of our conversation or if he had accepted his fate with relief.

The doctor asked, "John, what has led you to choosing an accompanied suicide?"

"Because I am declining. My brain is losing the ability to function and without my brain I am not me. I do not wish to live in a chair drooling by a window."

"Is this something you recently decided or have you thought about it before?"

I worried, *Please John, don't say you don't want to be a burden to anyone. That will get you rejected. Please remember what I kept telling you. Worrying about being a burden means you are being influenced by outsiders. It has to be your choice alone. Please remember.*

"Oh, Erica and I have talked many times about what we'd do if one of us got Alzheimer's. We discussed it when we were younger. Erica's mother had early on-set Alzheimer's, so she had an upfront seat to the horrors of the disease. We did not know about accompanied suicide, but we knew we didn't want to live through to the end of it."

"Erica," the doctor asked, "so you are supportive of John's decision?"

"Yes, I am. But it is his decision."

Our doctor continued with his questions for about 45 minutes and then told us. "I will be able to send you this report within one week. I am sorry to meet you both under these conditions. I can tell you are clearly a lovely couple and my heart goes out to you. I do find that you, John, have the mental capacity to make this decision on your own."

That was it. We were done. Until Switzerland.

Our Last Night

July 20, 2023

I had a dream last night—actually it was more like a visitation.

John was walking on a mountain road alone and came upon Methuselah. Methuselah was dressed in a long robe and held a cane. Methuselah asked John, "Can I help you?"

John said, "Yes, I am looking for a specific address in Paradise."

Methuselah said, "Oh that is easy. I can help you find that."

I woke up with a feeling of warmth and peace and love. It gave me hope that John would be okay.

July 22, 2023 was a Saturday night. It was our last night together in San Francisco. We were leaving for Zurich the next day. I had already packed our clothes for our trip. I used a small carry-on for my clothes and put a few of John's things in it too. I put the rest of John's toiletries and clothes in his backpack.

He asked me, "Why are you taking so much, and I am not?"

I felt so incredibly guilty for having a future, but he did not. I felt so full of remorse.

"Because I am going to Palatine afterwards. I am going to stay for two weeks."

We had had this same conversation many times over the past few weeks.

I asked, "Does this bother you?"

He told me, "I am glad you are going to be with Dan and his family."

I asked John, "What would you like to do tonight, honey?'

"I don't care, Erica. What do you want to do?"

"Well, would you like to go to a movie? Maybe get a burger at Causwell's and see a movie on the street?"

"Ya, that sounds good. What's playing?"

"We are lucky. There are two good movies. We can see either Barbie or Oppenheimer."

"Ugh, I don't want to see Barbie. Let's go see Oppenheimer,"

"Are you sure? Oppenheimer will be heavy, and Barbie will be fun and pink."

"Yes, I am sure. I have zero interest in seeing Barbie."

"Okay, that's fine. I want to see both. I know Oppenheimer is supposed to be really good."

We walked hand in hand the four blocks to our favorite burger place. We always held hands when we walked anywhere. We held hands in the movie theater, the opera, the ballet, and often in the car while John drove. It was just natural. It was what he did.

The movie was excellent. We talked about the movie on our way home, holding hands. As we talked, I kept wondering if John was thinking that this was the last time he'd walk down Chestnut Street with me. I wondered if he thought about how this was the last time he'd pass by the Apple Store, Walgreens, the Marina Market, The Coffee Roastery, our favorite coffee shop, and all the other spots we have been going to for thirty years.

I didn't ask him.

John's Wallet

I had to take his credit cards and his driver's license away from him. I took his watch and wedding ring. John watched me. He watched me empty his wallet of his valuables and his money. He asked, "Don't you just want to take the whole wallet?" "No," I answered impatiently. "I don't want the wallet!" I was wiping out his life and he calmly watched me do it. Did I make him sad? I'll never know. Could I have cleaned him out in a different way? Could I have talked to him more about it? Could I have been gentler—less distressed? Could I have been more?

I felt like a warden in a prison. I was his wife—his loving wife of forty-one years and I was methodically separating him from his life. I kept wondering how he felt, but talking didn't feel right. John was so compliant. He slipped off his ring. He calmly searched his wallet for all I needed and then looked at me with those beautiful blue eyes—eyes that smiled at me—eyes that have always made me smile. He was ready to go.

My Charm Bracelet

In high school in the early 1960s, bobby socks and saddle shoes were our uniforms, but when we got dressed up, charm bracelets on our wrists were our fashion statements. Everyone had a gold charm bracelet that dangled small meaningful trinkets for each girl.

My mom gave me mine one Christmas. I was delighted. It came with one charm on it, a tiny, graceful ballerina because I was a ballerina. As birthdays and Christmases piled up, so did my charms. My parents and brothers all gave me charms symbolic of my life and my heart's desires.

We lived on a cul-de-sac in a lovely Chicago suburb in a large three-story Tudor home. My parents had decorated our side with a lantern light to show our address across the top just like a street sign: 450 Lakeside Place. One of my favorite charms was a miniature of this. If I pushed the bottom, it lit up just like the one on our street.

My bracelet boasted a bejeweled charm with "Sweet 16" engraved on the front and a small gold box with a dollar bill stuck inside. Two of my favorites were simple gold discs with my brothers' names on one side and their birthdays on the other.

When Jim died at thirty-three, I took his disc off the bracelet, bought a nice gold necklace, placed the disc on the chain, and wore it near my heart. I repeated that process when Terry died in 2010. I have worn that necklace with my brothers' discs close to my heart every day since.

I had no idea John noticed my gold chain with my dead brothers' names hanging from it. Perhaps, years ago I told him about it. I talked to John about Jim and Terry a lot. John was great friends with Terry, but, sadly, never knew Jim. But John knew how much I loved both of them and the simple ritual of wearing their discs around my neck made me feel closer to them. Often, I reach up to touch the discs. It is a catalyst to think about Jim and Terry.

John and I were in the kitchen one day not too far away from the day he would die. He stood in front of me, holding my necklace in his hands, and looked into my eyes. "Are you going to make one of these for me when I die?"

I was stunned and saddened. Without a blink. Without any hesitation. "Of course."

I don't know what he was thinking when he asked me. Did he think I would forget him? Was he just curious? Did he want to be included in my memorial around my neck because he didn't want to be left out? I don't know and it does not matter.

I think it was one of the sweetest and saddest things John has said to me. He was thinking about my life after his death. I feel sad that he thought about not being here with me anymore, but of course, he must have had those thoughts. I wish we would have talked more about life after he died.

I don't like thinking about John being sad. It breaks my heart and I feel guilty. But, realistically, how can one expect someone who is about to die to not feel sad?

When I was able to move my body again after he died, I went to a jeweler. It was my first act of my afterlife. I asked the jeweler to make a gold disc with "John" written on the front and 11-16-45 on the back in the same font and size as Jim's and Terry's.

Now I wear three discs around my neck. I touch three charms. Three gold memorials to those I love. They are near my heart—in my life and in gold.

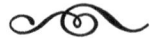

Gone With The Wind

I lost his ring
On my finger
I should have known
It could not linger
Maybe it returned to him
My finger was just too slim
Sadness overtook me
I no longer wore John
Looking for where it could be
Giving up to the fates that took his body
That took his brain
His ring has gone just the same.

Hotel Boldern

I wasn't sure my legs would walk me down the airplane gangplank. But John held my hand and I trudged along until we found our seats. I looked at our seats and said, "I think we are in the wrong section. This looks like Business Class."

John checked the numbers and said, "No, these are the right numbers."

Leave it to the one with Alzheimer's to figure out what seats we belong in.

We landed in Zurich on our last flight together.

John had slept some, but I can never sleep on an international flight. My body fights time zones as though my internal clock runs only on Pacific time.

We had no luggage to retrieve. We were traveling light. This was July 23, and I would be leaving Switzerland on July 26.

John only needed a backpack for his short stay. I obsessed about his backpack, making sure he had what he needed and yet could squeeze it all in. I bought him new soft sweatpants to wear on July 26 along with one of his championship Warriors t-shirts. I carefully folded them and then stuffed them into the backpack.

Nothing I did made any sense.

A taxi drove us to our hotel. I had picked the hotel from a list provided by Dignitas. John said, "Erica, we just spent $75 on a taxi ride! That's outrageous."

I thought, "Why does he care what we spend?"

The hotel sat right in front of Lake Zurich backed up by the Swiss Alps. It was a long ride from the airport, and I recognized nothing. John kept asking, "How far are we going? Where are we going?" I wondered the same. I had no answers.

The taxi delivered us to a low modern building with glass windows around the front. John and I looked at each other with curiosity; where is Zurich? The hotel's address is Zurich. John and I had traveled to Zurich on a few occasions; it is a big city with churches with spires and a big commercial shopping district. It boasts a lovely old town and lots of tourists and restaurants and a bustling financial district. "This must be somewhere else."

We walked into the empty lobby in the early afternoon. One receptionist checked us in and told us where our room was.

"Hello," she greeted us. Welcome to the Hotel Boldern. Welcome to Zurich. You are checking in?"

John stood next to me as I handled the check-in process. "Thank you. Yes, we are checking in."

"May I have your last name and your passports, please."

"Of course, Baccus is our last name and here are our passports. I also want to let you know our son will be checking in tomorrow."

"Thank you. As you can see the dining room is right behind my desk -the big room with the glass windows. Your room will be 229. Just take the elevator around the corner on the right and get off on the second floor. This key will unlock the door for you. How many keys do you need?"

"We'd like two keys. Can you tell me what time dinner is?"

"Dinner starts at 5 PM. You will not need reservations. We are not fully booked. Let me give you your passports back. Thank you and enjoy your stay. We are happy you have arrived safely."

There were no people in the lobby or the large dining room which faced the lake and the mountains. John looked out the window and asked me, "Are we in Costa Rica?" I looked at him not knowing what had just happened. "No, honey, we are in Switzerland."

I had arrived in the world of the absurd.

The lobby and the dining room were large rectangular rooms which could have been the site of a conference room in an airport or hotel in anywhere, USA. There were cows roaming the grassy area outside with bells around their necks. A house speckled the landscape here and there, but I saw no hiking trails, no shops, no sign of life except the cows. I asked the receptionist, "What do people do here?" She answered with no irony, "Nothing."

I sank and sank. It started to rain. I was exhausted. Maybe our room would lift my spirits. We walked into a small dark room with a bed stuck in the middle and a desk against the wall. There was hardly room to put even the backpack on the floor. A closet opened into the room stuck between the bed and the desk and an extra chair sat next to the desk.

I turned on a light which made almost no difference. That room is burned into my brain. It was so depressing and so the opposite of what we needed. This room is where reality started to hit me.

The whole hotel reeked of sadness, and the room was the worst. It was the place where my emotions started to crawl out of the cage I had locked them in.

John and I looked at each other and I asked, "Do you want to take a nap?" Sleep seemed like the most rational thing to do. We crawled into our low narrow bed, cuddled up and pushed reality from our consciousness.

Day 2: July 25

Thunderstorms continued so we could not even take a walk outside. It was just a waiting game to say the last "I love you."

I asked John, "Do you know how deeply I love you?"

"Yes, I do."

Dan arrived in the late morning. He brought vitality with him. Pressure moved from me to him. He would help the hours be more comfortable.

John and Dan played pool. They laughed. I watched and marveled at the normalcy. I tried to stop time and failed.

Later in the afternoon, jet lag set in for all of us. We retreated to our rooms for a nap and set our alarms to wake up in time to meet the doctor who would be examining John.

The doctor appeared at our hotel room door early in the evening before dinner. Dan joined us in our room. There was room for the doctor and John to sit. Dan sat on the bed, and I found a corner on the floor where I could be comfortable.

If John failed this interview, we would be headed home. I was nervous and conflicted. We had no plans for failing—no plans for returning home with John. Yet, the doctor was so casual about the conversation, John forgot the consequences. The doctor wore jeans and a long–sleeve plaid shirt. He was short compared to John's almost six feet and Dan's six feet one inch. He was very friendly and put one at ease quickly.

"Hello, John," he said. "Please get comfortable and we can chat for a little bit. How was your flight?"

"The flight was long, but all went smoothly. No problems."

"So, John, I just want to ask you a few questions about why you are here and your intention for an accompanied suicide. Tell me a little bit about your illness."

"Well, I have Alzheimer's and I know it's getting worse. I can't remember anything. I use Erica's brain to help me get through each day."

"I understand," the doctor went on. "You know you don't have to decide today that you want to do the accompanied suicide. You can go home and come back anytime you want."

"No, I want to do this now. I am losing my brain, and I don't want to live like this. If I don't have my brain, then I am not a person. My brain is who I am, and I do not want to exist in this world without it."

I have heard this speech several times before. I felt relieved he remembered not to say he didn't want to burden his family. I remembered how this would kill his chances.

"I have thought about this for a long time, and this is what I choose to do. I am not afraid to die. I have had a wonderful life and now it is time for me to go. I am grateful for all I have experienced in my life, and I have no regrets."

I was grateful for his positive attitude. I still needed reassurance that this was the right thing to do.

The doctor shook hands with us all and quietly left us in the room together. He told John, "I'll be back in the morning at breakfast to have one last conversation with you, John. You can sleep on your decision."

John said to me, "Erica, my time is running out. You know if I waited any longer, I would soon not be able to pass the mental capacity test. I would not be able to have that conversation with the doc."

"I know, sweetheart. It's okay."

Dan, John and I went to have dinner in the large empty dining room whose glass walls elegantly looked out on Lake Zurich. I sat facing the lake with Dan next to me and John across from me. The rain had stopped. The thunder had quieted down. I looked up from my menu and saw a miraculous rainbow. The largest rainbow I had ever seen. It spanned the lake and the mountains full of every color in the rainbow and it stayed. "John," I quietly yelled, "look behind you. Look at this rainbow. It's amazing. Dan, hurry up and take some pictures."

I got my phone out to take photos and I kept wondering how long this rainbow would stay. Then, I felt a wash of peace slide over my body, and I took a deep breath.

That night, our last night, John fell asleep quickly. He was on his side with his back to me. I tried to spoon him. I whispered, "John."

I thought, *How does someone who knows he is going to die in the morning sleep so soundly?*

I lay awake wondering how my life, our life, could be ending like this.

Day 3: July 26

We both showered. I laid out John's new unworn soft sweatpants that I bought at Nordstrom for this day. I took a moment to remember my shopping trip.

I had parked my car in the mall lot and walked solemnly to the store. I entered and thought, *This is a bizarre shopping trip. What will I say if someone asks me what or who the sweatpants are for?* I knew, of course, there was probably no reason for anyone to ask that, but I was feeling very exposed. My emotions flooded to my mouth and heart. Tears clouded my sight. I asked a saleslady, "Where can I find men's sweatpants?"

"Over on the right towards the back."

"Thank you," I said. I found the department and again asked for help. "I need to buy new sweatpants for my husband. Can you tell me which brand is popular?"

With each step I took towards the men's section, I thought *I am shopping for clothes for John to die in. Not a birthday present. Not a Christmas present. But the last thing he will wear. This is so hard. This is weird.*

The lady showed me piles and I felt each brand seeking the softest, most comfortable ones. I thought, *I want John to feel good in these.* Then I thought, *Erica, you know you are not being rational.* But I didn't care. I wanted John to feel loved at the last moment and that I cared enough to buy him new sweats that were soft.

Returning back to the present, I handed him his favorite Warriors champion t-shirt. Then I collected all the rest of John's clothes and stuffed them into his backpack. John watched me. He asked no questions.

I left his backpack in a corner of the room for someone else. We met Danny in the dining room. I shall always remember the darkness of that morning and the heaviness in my heart. I shall always remember that I did what needed to be done while the saddest day of my life was beginning.

It is not normal to choose the date for your husband to die. It is not normal to orchestrate your husband's death. I wish he had died of a stroke or heart attack or cancer. I wish he'd gotten hit by a bus. I will be living with all of the complicated questions I have for the rest of my life.

As we sat at the breakfast table wondering what to eat, the doctor walked in and sat at our table. "Good morning," he said. "How did you sleep? Well, John, I told you I'd give you time to think about your decision. Have you changed your mind?"

Without hesitation, John answered, "No, I have not changed my mind. I told you yesterday this is what I need to do. This is what I want to do. This is my decision."

"Well, then. I approve your decision and you can continue the process. A car will be here in an hour to take you to the house. There will be two ladies there who will guide you through the process. I wish you well on your journey. Good-bye."

The car arrived on time and delivered the three of us to a house somewhere in Zurich. Two smiling middle-aged women greeted us outside. They escorted us into the house.

We could see one large room, but other smaller rooms existed behind these walls. The "kitchen" had a table and chairs while the adjoining larger area held a sofa, a reclining chair and a hospital bed off in the corner surrounded by windows.

We were asked to sit down and relax at the kitchen table. The ladies introduced themselves to us, but their names flew out of my brain. Who they were did not matter to me. They were part of the process, not my friends.

Lady #1: You can just sit here and chat for a while. I have called the police, and they will be here soon. "Why," I asked, "are the police coming?"

"Because they need to see John's face and match it to his passport. We need to ensure that John is John."

"Oh!"

John and Danny and I sat around a table waiting for the police to verify his identity. I have no idea what we talked about, but I know it was not important.

The police came relatively fast. "Who am I checking out?"

John said, "Me."

"Okay, then. I need to see your passport and driver's license."

I had John's passport which I showed to the police and John still had his driver's license, so he pulled it out. The police looked at the photos and matched them to his face.

"Thank you," he said, "good-bye."

Next, one of the ladies explained to us that John had to take an antiemetic drug so that he would not vomit up the medicine that would cause him to die. She said it would take half an hour to take effect.

She asked, "When would you like to take the antiemetic?"

"I'll take it now," John replied.

"Which chair or bed would you like to use?"

I popped up immediately, "I want to cuddle with John while he drinks the drink."

"Then, I recommend you choose the hospital bed."

We hung around the kitchen table until the lady said, "The half hour is over. The antiemetic will work now. You can get into the bed anytime you want now."

John stood up and I followed him. Dan disappeared into another room. John and I climbed into the hospital bed and he put one arm around me. The lady sat by his side in a chair with a lap full of Swiss chocolates. She explained, "The drug is very bitter. I can give you some chocolate to cover up the taste."

John had a small paper cup in his left hand and she filled it with the drug. He asked me, "Shall I do it now?"

I shrugged my shoulders.

John took a sip and with a smile he exclaimed, "Oh my god, this is awful. Is this the last thing I am going to taste before I die?"

The lady next to him answered, "No, I told you I have chocolates for you right here in my lap."

John reached his hand out for the unwrapped candy and stuffed about four pieces in his mouth at once. Then he finished his drink.

He lay down and spooned with me. He was behind me with his arm curled under my body. I could not see him but after about three minutes I felt his arm drop and my body fall onto the bed. I turned to look at him and he was asleep.

I sat up and put my hand on his heart until I could no longer feel it beat. I watched as his skin turned bluish white and then bluish purple. I asked the lady, "Is he gone? Is John dead?"

"Yes," she said.

"Can you check his heart with a stethoscope?"

"No, we don't have any here."

"I don't want to leave him until I know for sure he is dead."

"I can check his pupils for you with the penlight."

"Yes, please do." I watched his lovely blue eyes stay still. I knew his life had left him—left me. I sat by his bedside holding his hand.

Danny opened the door and came to the bedside. "He doesn't even look like John. That is not John."

I did not see what my son saw. I saw my dear husband laying lifeless on the bed. I knew I needed to leave him there, but I wanted to stay with him. It seemed cruel to leave John alone in a strange room with strangers. I also knew I was not being rational.

I leaned over his bedside to give John one last kiss good-bye. Then Dan and I left for the airport. I knew I was leaving my life behind me.

The Flight Home

I had to continue moving in the direction of getting the "green light," so John could die in peace. There was one more major task to complete before leaving the US for Switzerland, but I couldn't get myself to do it. I needed to make flight reservations for John, Danny and me to go to Switzerland and a return flight for just Danny and me. Just thinking about saying those words to a United Airlines person on the phone felt overwhelming and impossible.

I called Jacki, my friend and travel agent, on May 24. Jacki had known John's illness was accelerating, but she had no idea about our plan. I trusted Jacki to keep my confidence and to help me with compassion and no drama. Still, calling her out of the blue to ask her help was something I had to really think about.

I imagined the scene. "Hi Jacki. This is Erica. I need your help. John and I need to fly to Switzerland in July so he can die. Can you make the reservations for me?" *Good God. How do I do that to her? And then ask her not to say anything to anyone else.*

That is basically what I did.

"First, I am going to tell you something very sad. Also, I am asking that you do not tell anyone about this conversation. I really need you to keep this confidential for a number of reasons. Jacki, John has decided he wants to end his life on his own terms. He does not want to live through the end of Alzheimer's. We have found a place in Switzerland where he can participate in what they call an assisted suicide. We need to go to Zurich in July, but I find that I cannot make the reservations. Can you help me?" I got it all out as fast as I could. Rip the Band-Aid off.

"Oh my god, Erica. I am so sorry. I had no idea. Of course, I'll help you and I promise this is between us. You don't have to worry about that. Can you give me the specifics so I can get to work on this?"

"Yes, John and I need to fly from San Francisco to Zurich to arrive on July 24. I need a flight for Danny to fly from Chicago to Zurich to arrive on July 25. Then Danny and I will fly home to Chicago on July 26. The thing is John is going to die on July 26 and I want to get out of Switzerland as soon as possible. I don't want to spend the night there. So, we will need a flight late in the afternoon."

"Okay, do you know when you want to come back to San Francisco?"

"No, not yet. I need some time to figure that out. Can I get back to you on that?"

Even more bizarre was the fact that I had to email Dignitas to confirm the schedule for John's death in order for me to figure out when I could logistically get to the airport on time for a flight. As I write this it feels as nuts today as it did then—just writing these words feels like an out of body experience. How on earth did I have the ability to plan these details?

I suppose my task mode took over. I made a promise to John and I needed to honor his wishes.

I certainly did not want to rush the last moments we had together. I certainly knew I wanted to spend as much time with him as he wanted—as I wanted. I knew that once he drank the drug, it would take effect in about five minutes.

Jacki had a difficult time finding a flight for Dan and me, but she succeeded. It would be tight depending on what time we actually left for the airport, but she was pretty sure it would all work out.

Dan and I left the Dignitas house early enough to arrive at the airport on time. I had one foot out the door of the limo and he was standing at my door to help me out. He had his phone in his hand, and he said, "Mom, our flight has been canceled."

Sometimes life is just not fair.

The Unexpected Overnight

I was exhausted, nervous, and probably in some kind of shock. First, I needed to find a new flight. I met with a lady at a special desk. She was kind and efficient. But John had just died an hour ago and making airline reservations felt absurd.

"I'm sorry. There are no flights to Chicago any longer today."

"What? You mean no airlines at all?"

"There is one flight you can take to Frankfurt today and spend the night there. Then take an early morning flight to Chicago. But I have only room for one person."

"That doesn't help. I want to leave for Chicago today. I don't want to be separated from my son."

"Let me look again."

It seemed to take a very long time. She typed and typed. I have often wondered what these airline reps are doing when they type forever. I waited with my head in my hands while Dan stood behind me quietly.

"I am so sorry for the inconvenience, but the only flight I can find for both of you leaves tomorrow morning. It goes non-stop to Chicago and has the Premier Economy you paid for."

"Okay, we will take this. Thank you. What do we do now?"

"I can give you vouchers for the hotel, food and shuttle to and from the airport."

"Thank you very much. You have been very helpful."

I was numb.

Dan and I picked up our carry-ons and walked over to the shuttle. The hotel seemed nice enough. It was now 4 p.m. and I had not eaten anything since dinner the night before. We were both hungry and walked into the dining room. The dining room was closed until 7 p.m. Not even a vending machine with Snickers was available.

"What do you want to do, honey?" I asked.

"Let's just go to our rooms. Maybe we can take a nap."

Danny's room was next door to mine. He opened his door and said, "Let's meet at 7 p.m."

I tried to watch TV but couldn't focus. I fell asleep immediately. Danny knocked on my door around 7 p.m. We took the elevator to the dining room level and found a table. We barely spoke.

We returned to our rooms after dinner and agreed on a time to meet to leave for the airport. I could not sleep. I could not cry.

At 2 a.m. I heard my text sound. I picked up my phone and read the text. "Mom, are you awake?"

I texted back. "Yes, I am."

"Do you want me to come in there?"

"Oh my gosh, yes, please!"

I opened my door and my son walked in. "Danny, will you lay down in bed with me?" He lay down and let me put my arm around him from behind. The comfort of his body—the comfort of knowing he was with me let me give in to my exhaustion. I fell soundly asleep until the alarm went off in the morning. This was probably one of the kindest gestures anyone has ever done for me. I shall always be grateful for his compassion.

Some sort of extreme exhaustion set in. I could not walk through the airplane terminal without stopping several times. "Mom, are you okay?" I wondered what was wrong with me. My legs just wouldn't work, and I had no idea why not.

"Yes, I just need to rest a bit. Give me a minute."

As we waited for departure, Dan went to get water and some snacks. He left me at a table. When he returned, I was fast asleep with my head on the table.

Finally, it was time to board the Swiss Airlines flight to Chicago. The gate clerk stopped me just as I was getting ready to walk the gangway and said, "Ms. Baccus, you have been bumped to Business Class."

"I have? Pointing to Danny behind me, I asked, "Is he bumped also, because I am not going without him."

"Yes, you are both in Business Class."

Finally, that angel who is supposed to sit on my shoulder showed up. I have no idea why we were upgraded. I have just accepted it as a gift. Was it from John?

The Sunroom

It is the smallest room in our house. But we spent most of our time in the sun-room. It has a southern exposure, giving us all kinds of light during the day. Out the window, I can see the San Francisco streets as they go uphill from my flatlander home. Our garden looms three stories below, showcasing its plum and cherry trees, lilies and agapanthus and homegrown vegetables. Most importantly I can see two chairs on the patio John built. I can see where John sat to rest when he tired of gardening and the chair saved for me when I went out to sit by him.

Our cat, Felix, sits on the edge of the sofa warmed by the sun. He too looks out the window. Maybe he eyes the birds and the butterflies or maybe he watched John too. John was his person, so it mattered where John sat.

I went to the window often during the day to see how he was doing. Was he asleep in the sun or climbing a ladder that I wished he didn't climb to reach a high limb? Was he pruning the bushes or watering the plants or sitting and memorizing his sanctuary?

I look out the window now and it all seems so empty. I try so hard to make it matter, but all I see are empty chairs and no reason to leave my house.

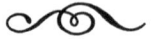

Hope

I collect hope stones
Hoping to find hope
What will it look like
When hope is near
How will I know I have hope
Slipping through my fingers
Fragile to hold on to
Sometimes a moment
Feels good
Sometimes a thought
Tells me it's okay
And then it is gone
I shall keep looking
For more hope stones
Maybe one day
I will find the right one

Good-bye Letter

How on earth do you tell everyone you care about, everyone you have dinner with, everyone you play golf with and ski with, everyone who has been your friend for forty years that you have suddenly left them forever? I borrowed from Amy Bloom and decided to send an email out on the day John would die. I knew it would come as a shock. I knew some would be angry or hurt or just desperately sad. But it seemed the best way for John and me and the best way to let everyone know at once.

Jennifer, my loving and very reliable friend, promised me she would send out our email on the appointed time and day. I gave her my contact list and she dutifully hit send on the morning of July 26.

Dear Friends and Family,

Some of you know and some of you do not. John was diagnosed with Alzheimer's Disease in January 2020. It has been a difficult, demanding and heartbreaking time and through it all three things have been unwavering: our love for each other, our loving and supportive families and John's clear decision that he would not and did not choose "the long goodbye" of Alzheimer's over the next many years.

A Promise Kept

John loved his life, his family and his friends. He loved his garden and his train and his hacker golf scores. But, in his words, he could not bear to be a living corpse. He believed if one could not give back in life then it was not a life he wanted. So, together we made arrangements to end his life peacefully, painlessly and humanely at Dignitas in Zurich, Switzerland with me by his side.

John remained loving and funny, brave and accepting of his fate throughout the last seven months of planning and preparing. He tried to continue to live the best life he could and was committed to making sure I knew how to plant tomatoes.

The Celebration of Life will be held at the Golden Gate Yacht Club on September 9 at 1:00 PM. John's family and I would be very happy to have you join us to say a proper farewell to my loving husband.

A formal invite will be sent to you in the near future.

Love to you all, Erica

Planning The Memorial

"Honey, what kind of memorial would you like me to have for you?"

"I don't need you to do anything."

While the celebration of life was all about John, it was for me. John knew I needed friends and family to come together to help me say good-bye to him.

"Have a picnic in a park somewhere. Maybe on Chrissy Field."

"John, it's too hard to have a private event in a public park. Never mind. I guess I will figure it out."

I felt odd planning John's memorial in early June while he was still alive. I did not speak about it to John ever again. It felt very weird to me, but I needed to have something ready. I was used to the traditions of the Jewish religion where the funeral is supposed to be held within forty-eight hours of the death. While I certainly wasn't trying to hold to those traditions, there was that part of me that felt like waiting many months after would not work for me.

I tried to think of a place John would like. I had been to a memorial service at the St. Francis Yacht Club, and it was a lovely spot with its glass windows all facing the San Francisco Bay. I walked over there one day and asked about their availability, and they had none within the next six months. I had doubts about it anyhow, because it is an expensive, high-end, fancy club that John would not like.

I walked out of the yacht club into the parking lot and met my next-door neighbors coming in.

"Oh, hi, Erica. Are you here for an event?"

"No, I said. "Why are you here? Are you members here?"

"No, Dori said, we are here for our St. Ignatius reunion lunch."

"Oh, that's nice. Have a good time. See you later."

I wanted out of there fast. I felt like a criminal skulking around. They didn't know how sick John was. I couldn't possibly tell them I was trying to rent a room for John's memorial when he was sitting in the backyard. But the experience gave me an idea.

For many years John played golf with his friend Joe every Thursday. Joe belonged to the Golden Gate Yacht Club up the road from the St. Francis. So, every Thursday after golf Joe and John had drinks at the bar at the GG Yacht Club. They were regulars. They had their special seats at the bar. It was their Cheers bar. They knew everyone who came in and they stayed until 7 p.m. when Joe had to go home for dinner. On rare occasions I joined them, so I had a feel for the friendly ambience and rituals they so enjoyed.

I walked out of the parking lot and called the Golden Gate Yacht Club to set up a meeting with the manager. My first meeting was an introductory one so I could evaluate the club's appropriateness for the memorial.

Bob, the manager whom I recognized, greeted me at the door and invited me to sit down.

"I'd like to talk to you about renting your space for an event."

"Let me give you a brief overview of how we work."

"Perfect."

When he was done explaining how the seating, food and bar worked, he took me for a tour of the room. The main hall sits on the San Francisco Bay with windows all around. The view of the Golden Gate Bridge is seen from every possible table, and it's spectacular. I could see Sausalito, Tiburon, and Alcatraz. Down a few steps was a bar and place for appetizers. This was not the same room where John sat every Thursday but similar. I heard John in my head say, "Do a picnic in the park." This was the park, and I could serve an elegant picnic.

Bob then invited me to sit down to talk about details. "What kind of event are you hosting?"

I held back my tears, "It's a memorial service."

"Oh, I am so sorry, Erica."

"Thank you."

"About how many people would you expect to attend?"

"I am not sure. Maybe around fifty. How many people can you handle here comfortably?"

"Fifty is perfect. We can manage about 100 people if necessary." When are you thinking of doing this?"

"Do you have availability in September?"

"Yes, I do. We are booked towards the end of the month but have some openings earlier."

"That sounds good. Can I get back to you?"

"Of course." Bob walked me to the door. We said our nice to meet you and goodbyes.

I left feeling a sense of relief and extreme sorrow. I went home and looked over the material Bob had given me. I decided I would sign a contract after we had our next meeting to review more specifics.

I arrived on time for our next meeting feeling a bit nervous and self-conscious. Bob greeted me warmly and said, "Let's sit over here at this table. It has such a beautiful view. Erica, may I ask who this memorial is for?"

I was silent for a bit too long, because then Bob offered that I didn't have to tell him. But, I said, "It is for my husband, John Baccus."

"Oh my god. I didn't put your name together with him. I knew he was sick, but I did not know he died. I am so sorry, Erica. I really liked John. He was always so friendly and fun to be around."

"Thank you, Bob. John has not died yet. He will die in July." Then

I explained it all. Awkward, self-conscious, embarrassed and sad. I felt it all and realized how often I would have to go through this when friends found out.

Gretchen is one of my heroes. I returned to her house after Switzerland, and she knew how to let me grieve. She was kind and thoughtful but not full of pity. I asked her to help me create and send out invitations to the memorial service and to help me choose a menu.

Without any drama, Gretchen worked on both tasks and took over all the details of managing the invite; creating it, emailing it and recording RSVPs for me. I respect Gretchen's opinion on all kinds of things, but especially for event details. She helped me make all the small but important food decisions such as how many vegetarian options we needed, and what kind of desserts and how many main-course items we should offer.

Bob was gracious. He began by expressing his sorrow again and his understanding for me. He told me about his mother who went through the horror of a long death with Alzheimer's and supported our decision. He made me feel a bit less uneasy and hearing his story helped confirm the wisdom of our journey.

We worked together for the next few months, and he was always so kind. I was certain I had chosen the right place to honor John's memory.

The food was presented beautifully and more importantly it tasted good. I would not know, though, because I could not eat anything. The highest compliment came from Owen. "Grandma, most of the time funeral food is terrible. I loved your food."

A Promise Kept

Shortly after John died and I had returned home, I needed to create a program for the memorial service. Like most people, I started by Googling program templates for celebrations of life. Everything I saw made me want to vomit. The templates were either religious, sappy, not enough space for content or just plain ugly. I sat at my desk, head in hands, wondering what to do when suddenly I realized this program was just another book.

I have been making electronic books with my photography for our family for decades. I could make the program myself. I have eighty thousand photos on my computer so there is no shortage of photos of John and our family and friends. I had as much space as I needed for the program agenda and I could include poetry, personal comments from family and whatever else I wanted. Most importantly, I could make it personal—about John, and I knew my love would come through the pages. It turned out exactly as I wanted.

I asked our good friend, Jim, who is a talented creative director, if he could help me make a video of John for the celebration of life. Without hesitation, he told me he would be honored.

Now I watch the video and see John and me celebrating our lives each and every day. I am grateful for the video. I am grateful for the life John and I had.

John's Celebration of Life was held at 1:00 PM on September 9, 2023. It was a beautiful, clear- blue-sky San Francisco fall day. Ninety-three friends and family helped me say goodbye to my dear husband.

The Day the Ashes Came

I was doing something meaningless in the house when my doorbell rang. It rarely rings in the middle of the day. I wandered down the stairs, opened the door to a deliveryman who asked me to sign for the box he was holding. I was not expecting anything. I signed the form. He then handed me a large box and he left. I closed the door.

I looked at the label on top of the box and saw that it was sent from Dignitas in Switzerland.

I knew immediately it held John's remains. I just was not expecting this so soon. How efficient the Swiss are. It took me completely by surprise. Crumbling on the stairs crying my heart out, I called for my sister to take the box—to let her open it.

I have not yet touched the bag that holds his remains. It is hidden in his closet with shirts and towels covering it. I cannot look at the box that holds the bag. I am both repelled and shocked by it.

This is what is left of my dear husband's body. It is barbequed and gross. I find nothing sentimental or beautiful about it at all. We had talked about his cremation. He said I should toss him in the backyard. The garden he tended so well for so many years. He belongs in his garden—in his earth, but I can't do it. I cannot imagine celebrating by spreading ashes. Maybe one day but not yet—maybe never. I think he would understand.

Now I think of the fire that incinerated his beautiful body and I want to empty my lungs and my heart of all its tears. I want to hold John in my arms and keep him safe.

I want so many things that can no longer happen.

Journal Notes

November 15, 2023

Owen called me today to say "Happy Birthday" to Papa and see how I am doing. I had been having a hard day. It is the day before John's birthday and one week before Thanksgiving. I started the day by pulling out all my Thanksgiving recipes and menus. I just completely broke down. It is so painful to do this without John.

So, Owen's phone call was very well-timed. I started to cry on the phone, and I told him, "Owen, I don't want to cry in front of you. I am the grown-up, and you are the kid."

Owen said, "Go ahead, Grandma, cry. It is understandable. I am sad too and I really miss Papa. Sometimes, Grandma, there are worse things than death. For you, having to live without Papa is probably one of them."

"I am not sure why I am here, Owen."

"Because you have grandchildren and your son and family."

He let me talk about my sadness. I said, "Sometimes my pain is physical. I am so sad it physically hurts. When I exercise it feels better."

"That's because exercise releases endorphins."

We talked about how John didn't want to go through the pain of Alzheimer's and he didn't want me or Owen or his family to go through the pain of watching him decline. Then we talked about how his first year in college is going.

He is looking forward to going home for Thanksgiving.

I am grateful for his compassion. He is wise beyond his years.

Erica Baccus

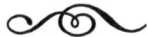

John's Birthday

Your birthday just passed
Where are you, I ask
I feel you within me
You are my guide
Nudging my side
I try not to mourn
Grateful you were born
How long shall you be gone
I'll wait for you
By the lemon tree

A Promise Kept

November 16, 2023

You gave me you. What more can anyone ask? I got you on the day we married, and you promised you would give yourself to me. For forty-one years, you gave me you. And you loved me as no one else could. I think that is pretty special. You are gone and I am here and I feel your arms around me. I feel your love.

It is your birthday today. It has been a hard day. I have tried to spend the time being grateful that you were born. I waited on this earth for almost two years for you to be born. Had you not been born; I would not have had the love that only you could give. I know no one who has loved as I love you or has been loved as I have. Nothing else matters. Not much more to say. We happened and I am grateful.

Erica Baccus

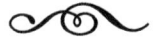

Absence

No tears for years
Now everyday
Joy has taken flight
I try with all my might
But he is gone away
And taken my smiles today
How shall I ever find peace
In a heart that is broken.
Joy
Comfort
Love
Safety
All gone
All lost

March 26, 2024

Today is seven months since John died. Grief overwhelms me, coming unannounced whenever it feels an opening. It feels heavy and unwelcome and carves holes filled with emptiness in my body. I have conversations with myself and with John. They are my "what-ifs." "What if you were still alive? What would you be like? What would our life be like?" Then I answer. "I don't care what you would be like. I just miss you. I just want you here."

People tell me to be grateful for the life we had. I am grateful, I think. But I am envious of my past life. I want to live it again. One of the most difficult phases of grief is not only mourning my loss of John, but my loss of a life I had lived for so many years. I would need to give up the familiar comforts of the life we had carefully created together.

I fear the future. I want to stop time, for I do not want to get too far away from when John was alive. I want to keep him near me. I want to keep us near me. I fear the spring when the weather gets nice. It starts the season of togetherness outside. I fear April for our next anniversary will arrive without him. Will I add a year to our marriage? I fear the summer, for it will bring me closer to reliving his death.

When John was alive, I was losing him and I missed him. When he died, I missed his aliveness. It is all perspective.

Today I learned, finally, how to put my Cuisinart together, so I could use it. I always had to ask John to assemble it. I am learning how to survive on my own. I don't like it.

May 2024

I am writing this nine months after I have lost my beloved. I spent most of my youth and middle age exclaiming I did not know if there is a god, or an afterlife. I was comfortable in my agnosticism. It was a middle ground that caused no conflict when those discussions arose.

Now I am no longer living this philosophical dilemma in theory. I am living it in reality. I do not know if there is a god. I shall not know this in my lifetime on this earth. But here is what I do know.

John's burned body is sitting in my closet, but I can feel him in spite of those ever-present ashes. His life touches mine. I can feel the whispers of his fingers on my arm. I can sit in a chair in his garden and conjure him into my space. His voice is soft-spoken, but we can talk to each other. I can hear him. Perhaps this is because he is so recently gone, but I choose to believe it is because his energy—his spirit—his humanity is with me or within me. Contrary to my unexplored and innocent beliefs, I now think quietly to myself that John lives within me. There is a part of him that has become me.

Tonight, I started to speak and I needed to stop. I thought, "The next words I shall speak are John's words. I am channeling him."

He said through me, "Owen, give yourself a break. Pat yourself on the back and accept your successes. You did great your first year in college."

I cannot and will not pretend expertise in this matter of belief. I will comfort myself in the knowledge that just as John promised, he is here with me. All I need to do is think about him and his presence is known to me.

Life After

July 29, 2023

I had a dream that I was sleeping in bed and someone was rubbing my shoulder. I was getting irritated. Then I heard John's voice asking me, "Don't you want me to do this? Should I stop?" When I realized it was John I said, "Yes, please go on. Don't stop."

August 31, 2023

It has been six weeks now since my life changed forever. I did not want this change. I miss John more than I could have imagined. Sometimes when I think about him my whole body hurts in a way I have never felt before. I really do not understand how I am supposed to move forward. The moment I think about John I start to cry. I would give anything for more time with him—even five minutes. Just five more minutes to have him hold me. To tell me I'm going to be okay.

Sometimes I think he was upset with me when he died. Sometimes I think I didn't show my love well enough. Sometimes I think I could have done a better job discussing the pros and cons of our decision. Sometimes I think I just didn't help him enough. Sometimes I think I was just in too much of a "let's get the job done" mode. Task-oriented, detached, unemotional.

Do I believe he was ready for this? Do I believe he was at peace with his decision? Do I believe he wanted to die instead of live with Alzheimer's, or was he just trying not to be a burden for me or anyone else?

I would give anything to do the last two days over again. I would have cried with him. I would have wrapped myself up in him and told him over and over again how much I loved him. Maybe I did and I don't remember. I was so jet-lagged, I don't remember much about those last two days. We slept a lot—did we cuddle and spoon? I don't recall. I do remember I tried to cuddle with him on his last night and he slept so peacefully and so hard that I could not disturb him. I recall thinking to myself; *how can anyone sleep like that the night before he is going to die?*

Perhaps Alzheimer's had something to do with it.

So now, I am interviewing gardeners, getting new locks on all the doors, trying to blow away the leaves, watering the garden and picking tomatoes. All things John used to do. In some ways, I feel closer to John when I work in the garden. But in some ways, doing his tasks makes me so aware that he is not here. I admit I have yelled at him a few times in the backyard. "Why, aren't you here? I don't know how to keep the grass green."

I don't mind being alone during the day. What makes me so inconsolable is not having John here to love me. I miss his smile, I miss hearing him say my name, I miss his arms around me, I miss his jokes, I miss his body and his company. I miss talking to him about everyday things and I miss hearing John say, "I love you."

I do not know how to get through this. I am not sure I want to get through this. I have a hard time grasping that this happened to us, because it was not supposed to. We were going to be very old together and have fun and love each other for a very long time.

I want my old life back.

Afterword

John and I are each in our own afterlife. His is a mystery to me and mine is a day-by-day exploration of how to survive separated from him.

It has been eight months now since he chose to leave for his journey. I have read the grief books, listened to meditation podcasts, talked to a therapist every week and cried on the phone to my very patient son and sister. The books warn that grief comes in waves and when it is least expected.

I have cried on the golf course, at the bank, on top of a ski mountain, in my car, at my desk, in my bed, in John's garden, in the cereal aisle at the grocery store, at the Thanksgiving dinner table, during Christmas present openings, and on the phone with my writing coach.

Sloane Crosley says in her book, *Grief is For People*, "I'd spent no small amount of time daydreaming how luxurious it would be to prepare for loss. Turns out the prepared version is not so hot."

When I read that sentence, I almost laughed. In one sentence Ms. Crosley aptly described my whole book. The thing is you can call knowing ahead of time being prepared, but there is no way to prepare one for the emotions that arrive afterwards. There is no way to prepare yourself for losing the person who always had your back, who cheered for you on the golf course, who loved your cooking, who dried your back when you got out of the shower, who jumped up and down with you when the Warriors won, and who spooned you every night.

I didn't think about how I didn't know how to put air in the tires, pay the taxes, wax the kitchen floor, put the Cuisinart together, fold the sheets alone, or fix a clogged sink.

There is no way to prepare for the sudden overwhelming depth of sadness that makes me wonder why I am here. Whose life have I impacted today?

I thank Owen many times a week in my head for giving me a reason to keep finding ways to make each day livable and worthy of my space in this universe.

I understand my pain will change. Hopefully, one day I will remember our love-filled, joyful, fun-filled life we had as Erica and John with a smile rather than pain.

But even now, I thank my dear John for giving me a life where I felt valued, beautiful, smart, sometimes funny, worthy and loved.

What's It All About, Alfie?

I hadn't thought about what kind of life we were leading. I hadn't thought about how we, with our individual beliefs and personalities, are molded into our marriage. Mostly, we just lived our lives, but oftentimes expressed our gratitude for our good fortune.

There is something so special in being able to quietly think to yourself, "I am happy." I had the good fortune to recognize my own state of mind.

I was happy.

Now I look back and see that our marriage was made up of those things we held dearest in our hearts.

The most vital element was our commitment to love each other. We had our struggles like most couples do, but we learned to work through them, to allow space for each other to be true to oneself, and to not give up. We had to learn to blend our families into one. Learning how to disagree was not easy. John wanted to escape a situation and I wanted to talk it over. Learning how to say "I'm sorry" was harder for John than me, but we both figured it out.

Love for us meant ensuring the other person was happy and our commitment meant that no matter what, we tried to find ways to help the other one be happy.

Our commitment to love meant I would help John die and do it without causing him guilt or suffering. Our commitment to love meant John would not have chosen this path had I objected and I knew that. Our commitment to love meant we both knew and accepted the other person's sacrifice. Our commitment to love meant that in the end we both knew we were loved fully and with joy.

Our marriage also endured loss. John chose a premature death, leaving me, his children, grandchildren and friends early. John lost time, which is all we really want. Family and friends lost time with John and I lost my life as I knew it.

But this wasn't our first loss. We both lost parents, brothers and first marriages in our lives that we took with us to our own marriage. We shared our grief. We shared our memories. Our past lives became part of our life together. We created an intimacy with each other that helped us through loss. When John chose his ending, he and I could talk about it honestly. He understood the overwhelming pain I would endure. I understood I needed to let him know I would be okay.

We were practical people. We both accepted what we could not change. I was motivated to get the job done and John was a believer in fate. Sometimes in our marriage these traits annoyed the other one; especially when I wanted John to change his behavior to help himself and he believed "I am who I am." John accepted his diagnosis with grace and an attitude of "I can't change this, so I need to accept it." I fed him blueberries and broccoli.

John taught me the importance of individual dignity and autonomy. Our forty-one years together were happy because John came to the marriage with the strong belief that each of us had the right to be—the right to be who we are. He helped me believe in my own independence so we grew to be two people who joined together in decision-making where appropriate, but also, we "did our own thing" without having guilt. John's decision to end his life on his terms was an extension of his autonomy, but it was a joint decision. It was not something he would have or could have executed without me as his willing partner.

Our love of family and our love for our family was constant and critical to our lives together. Vacations, holidays, phone calls and visits with family have always been at the center of our life together. During tough times we have given whatever we could to help. John and I believed in *family first*.

I saved the best for last. Having fun with each other was always present in our union. John was a fun person. He found joy in other people. He found joy in each day. He found joy in our life together. John made everything we did fun. When we first got married, he told me, "Erica, you are going to be bored with me after two years."

Nothing could have been further from the truth. I had so much fun with John that each day, each year was simply a good time. From the first time I heard his now-famous laugh I knew I wanted to spend time with this man who smiled exuberantly and who insisted life is supposed to be fun. His last words were a joke, "Is this the last thing I am going to taste before I die?"

Grieving

"I feel like I murdered my husband," I told my therapist.

Almost a year ago, John died of his own choosing. It has been a long and difficult time for me. John told me, "Erica, this is going to be harder for you than for me." I never responded to that. I did not believe him. He was going to die. I was going to live on.

But I think he was right. His death was his choice—not mine.

Writing our story has been healing for me. It has returned me to reality repeatedly, since I kept notes of what was *actually* happening during the last few years. To my surprise, after he died, I began to doubt our choices and my actions. I had spent most of my life over the past few years dedicated to taking care of whatever needed taking care of and helping John get approval from Dignitas. I did not allow myself to think beyond the day of his death.

I did not think about how I would feel. I did not let myself see what the loss of his presence would mean to me.

I understand that millions of women become widows and their lives are undeniably changed. They have to learn to adjust to their loneliness and loss of their normal life. They have to accept that their other half is missing. However, I do believe that the kind of death John chose has caused me to experience a different and additional kind of grief.

I write this not to complain or scare anyone away from assisted suicide. On the contrary, I am an advocate for assisted suicide. As I have said, John died in peace, painlessly with dignity. I believe in eliminating his kind of suffering.

But I was left with doubt. I struggled with, *Did I choose the right time? Could he have lived a few more months—maybe more?*

I beat myself up with, *Maybe I should have objected to his choice? Maybe because I did not object he thought I wanted him to die. Maybe because I did not object, he thought I thought he would be a burden? Maybe he wanted me to say, 'please don't'.*

I persevered on *Maybe I brainwashed him. Maybe it was my idea.*

I am just now recovering from guilt and unexplainable, unreasonable, irrational thoughts. They still overcome me at times. But now I have the ability to recognize these ideas are not based in reality.

I have listened to his videos where he has said, "Don't be sad for me. I am not sad for me. I have had a great life. Thanks to you, Erica. You have always made everything so special." I know these words by heart, because I have listened to him over and over again saying this.

I have read the book I wrote where I quote him saying, "Just shoot me, Erica. Just shoot me, now."

Had John been stricken by a heart attack or cancer or any other typical life-ending disease, I can imagine accepting it as a matter of fate. Tragic, maybe, sad, for sure. But not something that would cause the enormous guilt I have felt.

I orchestrated his death. I felt responsible for his death until I remembered it was Alzheimer's that was killing him. I went round and round in circles in my head thinking, *I did it*. and then I'd think, *No, it was Alzheimer's*. Then, *He chose to end his life*.

My new therapist is a wonderful psychiatrist who has been so helpful to both of us. He conducted John's last mental capacity exam before we went to Dignitas. He declared John capable of making his life-ending decision. At that meeting, I said to him, "I know that after this is all over, I am going to need some help. Are you able to take me on as a patient?"

"Yes," he declared. "My practice is focused on terminal patients and their caretakers. I would be happy to help you."

He is teaching me to see the other side. "If you had objected to John's choice, perhaps you would have only made his life more difficult. Did you want that to happen?"

"Rather than murdering your husband, the way I see it, you gave him a gift of love with grace." It brings tears to my eyes when he suggests what I did was loving. He is right though. I helped John because John wanted to die and he needed me to help him. I wanted John to have what he wanted.

John had an anthem in our marriage. "I have the right to be me." He taught me to respect this belief system and if I crossed the line, he assuredly let me know. So, whenever John asked, "Erica, what do you want me to do?" I had to answer "John, honey, I cannot tell you what to do with your life. This is your choice. You cannot think about me."

It was hard because obviously I did not want him to die, but I did very much believe he had the right to choose.

This path fit John perfectly. We discussed it many times during our marriage and John always maintained he would rather die than be a brainless vegetable.

What I regret is how fast he drank the medicine on that last day. I have thought, "Why didn't I stop him for a bit? Why didn't I make him take more time? Why didn't I tell him again how much I loved him? Why didn't I do something?"

Instead, John held the cup of poison in his hand and asked me, "Should I drink it now?"

What did I do? I shrugged my shoulders.

Who does that? He was going to die and I shrugged my shoulders!

I have watched this scene play again and again in my head.

My therapist has suggested to me that John had a choice. He was in charge. He was ready to go. He had free will. He has suggested it was not my decision, but John's. That helps.

The real problem is I do not understand John's courage and commitment to die.

My therapist tells me many people feel an enormous sense of relief once this kind of decision has been made. They are relieved to be done with their suffering.

I am glad John is no longer suffering. But now I am.

Yes, I am still grieving and find myself in puddles of tears in weird places and strange times. Sometimes the grief is so physical that it hurts.

However, there are moments when I feel the light of hope. Deep in my heart I believe I will find my new person. I will find a different life that will be recreated again through love and joy.

That is what John wanted for me. I promised him I would go on with a happy life. I shall fulfill my promise.

In time.

A Promise Kept

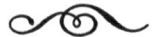

Weighing My Life

*I carry my grief with me
I carry my love with me
Unbalanced by my feelings
Split in two
Tears know no difference
The salt tastes the same
I am no longer whole
Broken apart by loss
Hope for stitching together
The torn seams of my life
Hope that one day
Love will weigh more than grief.*

Things I Wish I Could Ask John

1. Why are there fifteen very fresh, very crisp $100 bills in the poker case under the guest room bed?

2. What kind of bug is eating our rose bushes and what should I do?

3. Why do we have five sets of luggage stashed away in various closets?

4. Why didn't you live long enough to see me hit my drives one hundred fifty yards and break 100?

5. Why are there two boxes of rolled pennies, quarters, dimes and nickels under the bed?

6. Why does Felix meow at me in the middle of the night—every night?

7. Why do you have so many jackets and what should I do with them?

8. How should I pick the plums from the top of the tree?

9. Why does the TV set in the kitchen only get one channel?

10. Where did you go? Are you okay?

Appendix

Speeches From John's Memorial

My Comments

After I introduced our family and thanked everyone for coming; some from far-away places like Costa Rica, Denver, Wisconsin, Kansas City, Tahoe City, Illinois and Iowa, I talked about John and me and then our decision.

Not long ago John and I were discussing our love for each other. I told John his love for me made me feel valued and worthy, smart and beautiful and sometimes even funny. It was not from the words he spoke but from how he treated me. This was just how he made me feel.

There were so many ways I could have missed out on this fun-filled, love-filled, joyful and thoughtful journey. I am so grateful to fate for making sure I got on board for the glorious ride that was in store for me. I should also thank my son who at 14 said to me, "Mom, call John." The right words at the exact right time. (A long story for another time.)

John always said yes to me. Yes, to our adventures in travel, yes you should start your own business and yes to living in San Francisco.

Yes, to Ted you can live with us in our home, yes to Anya you can live here, yes to Trevor you can live with us, yes to Anne you can live here, yes to Louise you can live with us, and of course, yes to Dan you can live here.

He said yes to me when I quit three jobs in a row each no more than three months long and yes to me when I said I needed to leave Boston and go back to California after an honest eighteen months of trying Boston. Yes, of course let's go backpacking and yes you can teach me to ski and yes let's go camping with four little kids every summer for many years. Yes, Erica I'd love to try the SF Opera and the Ballet. Let's get season tickets even though we lived in San Jose, and it was a long ride home at night. Our marriage was built on yes. Yes, I love you, and we loved each other hard and long, and always with enthusiasm and joy.

AND then at the end, I had to say Yes to him when he asked if I would support him in his desire to end his life on his terms. I said I would do all I could to help him choose his own end of life—Yes John, you can die on your terms with dignity and humility. Yes John, you can die with me in your arms loving you through your very last breath and onward.

I wanted to say a few words about our choice to go to Dignitas, because so many people have asked me about it and people are confused about what is possible and what is not.

1. It is not possible to use California's End of Life Option Act or Oregon's Right To Die law for patients with any kind of dementia.

2. California law requires two doctors to swear an oath that

you will die within six months and you are mentally capable of making your own decisions.

3. The only place in the world that helps dementia patients is Dignitas in Zurich.

So as has been said, John knew immediately he did not want to live through the long good-bye of Alzheimer's and we discussed everything we could think of that we could do legally so that he could have control over his life and death.

Then in May 2022, a therapist referred me to In Love, by Amy Bloom. I purchased it and read it once and then twice. It is a memoir of Amy Bloom's journey with her husband who was diagnosed with Alzheimer's. Their lives were very different from ours, but the essence of the story is thankfully relevant. Amy Bloom did all the necessary research to find out how and where someone with dementia could choose how and when to end their lives. The answer to the dilemma is with Dignitas in Zurich.

I knew I had been given a gift when I finished the book. It took me a while to tell John about it, but once I did, he wanted to follow the same path. We continued to live our lives knowing at some point we would need to begin the application process—but not yet.

One of the most difficult decisions we needed to make was when is the right time. Of course, by definition his death would be premature, but we were threading a needle to make sure we got as much life as we could without compromising his ability to make rational decisions.

I knew I desperately wanted John to be able to attend our grandson's high-school graduation on May 23 and he thankfully did. We had plans to travel to Egypt with friends in October, but I knew when I made the plans there was most likely no way we could actually go. I kept planning our life's events knowing in my heart that John would likely not be able to participate.

Choosing the right time was a moral, ethical, practical and emotional problem for the doctors and for us. Eventually, by April of this year it became clearer that we were running out of time. If we pushed it too far, John could miss the window when he would still have mental capacity and he knew that. He did not want to miss his window.

Without going into minute details, I worked on all the necessary documentation and arranged John's necessary physician appointments for the last seven months to get him approved as a viable candidate for Dignitas.

The medical appointments included two psychiatric evaluations that stated John had the necessary mental capacity to make this decision on his own—uninfluenced by me or anyone else, that he understood what he was undertaking and he could lift a glass and drink on his own. The second evaluation had to be no more than three weeks prior to the event.

I sent in materials via email and waited anxiously for approvals I did not want to receive but also needed. John was a perfect candidate. He received the Provisional Green Light in May. The absolute final green light would only happen after meeting with the doctor in Switzerland.

So, I finished the process with Dignitas. John was reevaluated by another psychiatrist for his mental capacity exam on July 10—the last step before we flew to Switzerland.

John accepted his fate with love in his heart for his family and friends and would want you all to know he appreciated his great life.

So much more to the story but I am going to close with this thought:

I hope what you all take from our story is that we all should have the right to die with dignity—humanely, peacefully, and pain-free. John was grateful to exercise his right. As John said to me, "We were so smart in how we picked the right date."

Kyle's Eulogy

Since this is a celebration of life I'm going to try and keep it light-hearted. Plus, if I start crying, I'll get all choked up and won't be able to speak. So, I'm just going to tell you a bit about what it was like to have John for a dad.

We did a lot of outdoor stuff. He took me camping a bunch and he would do all the work, which I later developed an extra appreciation for when I tried to go camping without him. It was so much more fun when HE set up the campsite and did all the cooking while I just explored the wilderness. Somehow, the breakfast he would make at the campsite was the best thing ever. We went on hikes and canoe trips and did a lot of fishing. He passed down to me a love of nature and I really appreciate that.

What didn't get passed down to me was how he seemed to never get embarrassed. On those same camping trips, he almost always wore a goofy hat. I don't mean a funny-looking hat. I'm talking about the Disney character, Goofy. It had the dog face, flappy ears, buck teeth and a giant bill. It was so embarrassing, and he wore it all the time. He loved it because the long bill provided a lot of shade and he needed that.

There were some great things about him not getting embarrassed. He was the dad going around to all the other campsites gathering up kids so we could get a big game of Kick the Can going and we ended up having a lot of fun with strangers. He never hesitated to chat up a stranger who got within shouting distance. He had such a great personality. They always seemed to enjoy talking with him. I love how he was always in a good mood and how his good mood was contagious to those around him.

Everyone seemed to love him, *uuuuunless* you were a subpar server at a restaurant. He liked to give them an earful. I remember, even at a young age, being aware of how many times the server made a mistake and I could tell at a certain point my dad had decided they were going to have a conversation. Lori would grab me before the bill came and we'd head outside to escape the embarrassment. I appreciate that he was honest and let people know how he felt, good or bad.

As a kid, having John for a dad was kind of like having a really fun, silly friend that was always in a good mood and had great ideas for fun things to do. PLUS, he could drive a car and he paid for everything, and when we got in trouble with the grown-ups (Erica), he would take all the heat. It was great! We used to have sock fights! Inside the house! The rules were simple. Ball up some socks and throw them at each other! As you can imagine the adult (Erica) did not appreciate this! I was just a kid. Don't blame me, but I clearly remember when I would ask my dad to have a sock fight. It's like

I could see his thoughts as I patiently awaited his answer. I could tell he was conflicted, but almost always the kid in him would win out and socks would be flying!

I got to be on the other side of this equation when he would come to my house to visit my kids, so I sympathize with you, Erica, but seeing how much my kids loved playing with him like I did was wonderful. He was just as fun and energetic in his later years as he was with me.

My dad had such a joy for life, and he really was a kid at heart. I'm thankful he never grew out of that. He was so good at making things fun and would always come up with some little way to entertain me when things got boring.

What stands out to me the most about my dad is that I don't recall him ever being distracted or preoccupied. He was so good at being present and living in the moment.

My dad was really great with kids, but he also made a great adult. As I got older and started questioning how the world works, he was always my first call. He was a great person to get advice from or debate a topic with. It seemed like any subject I wanted to talk about, he had some useful knowledge of.

I'm really going to miss those conversations.

The last time I saw my dad we were talking about all the different possibilities of what could be waiting for us after this life. He told me he would try to make something move that shouldn't and to keep an eye out for it. Shortly after he passed, I was walking through Walmart in an empty aisle and a roll of bagels fell over as I walked by. What surprised me was how quickly I said "Hey Dad" out loud as it happened. Probably a coincidence I know, but it feels good to think that means everything is okay.

Dan's Speech

Lots of times I've been asked *what is a stepfather?* Many would ask if I ever called John Dad. Even after all these years, I'm not sure what a stepfather is.

I remember waking up early on school days and going off to school and John telling me to have a good day. I hated that, because I hate the mornings. I never said anything back to John, probably just grunted at him and wished he stayed quiet. But he always wished me a good day. Now, I do it with my kids.

In high school, I remember John teaching me to drive a stick shift and I remember him trying to teach me math. It was all bad. He was a bad teacher, but I was a worse student. But he was always willing to try another day.

I also remember in high school coming home and telling my mom and John that I ran a mile under seven minutes. John said he could beat it. He was so confident and sure he could beat my time. He started a typical family dinner argument and I bet him he couldn't beat my time. So, one weekend, we went to the local junior high… he completed half the laps and quit. As a teen, I looked at him and felt sorry for him. But now I know he was just trying to make things more interesting.

John made the best tacos. He fried the shells. Today I make my kids tacos, but I don't fry the shells. John was the kind of guy who took time to fry the shells.

He was the best at grilling. During the summers in Tahoe, I always looked forward to when John grilled steak. Soon, both Owen and Noah also loved his grilling too. John was happy to grill for us, of course. But I think one of his favorite parts of grilling was grilling on the public grills. There he would strike up a conversation with a stranger, tell his tales and laugh with complete strangers who had just become his best friend. He'd come back and tell us," I just met Joe and he was in the Navy in World War Two." To me it seemed like he just had the best time ever. I always wondered, "How did he do that?"

When Gretchen was on bed rest during her pregnancy, and we lived in the apartment underneath him, he came down once a week and cooked this fantastic fried chicken. My mom says it was her recipe and she always reminds us the recipe came from her. But to Gretchen and me, we know it as John's fried chicken.
When the boys were toddlers, John would take the boys on the train, or to the park or take them out to eat for breakfast. As the boys got older, he would play sock fights with them and a few years later he would wrestle, poke, prod, and yell with them. The boys loved the play fights and of course they loved him. And it seemed like the playing around would never stop. Finally, Gretchen or I would have to tell them to stop. I think John was the most disappointed.

Of course, John had wild and crazy ideas. He would always want to get in debates with me about sports. He loved the arguments. I think he just took the other side because it was more fun. Of course, if he heard me now, he would say that I was wrong and it wasn't true.

My uncle Terry and John were the first ones to take me to Reno when I was twenty-one. Then it became an annual tradition. But when John played Blackjack, he didn't care about winning. He only cared if he could get in a good conversation and talk to people at the table. After a while, you could hear his laugh around the casino.

One of my last memories of John was skiing with him this spring break. He was tired and wanted to go home so I said I would ski down the mountain with him. Because of his Alzheimer's, I begged him over and over again to stay behind and follow me. But true to his spirit, as we were going down the hill, John raced past me.

There are so many ways John was a part of my life. When I think about him lately, I can feel him. I see his shiny face and hear his hearty laugh. He was just such a good guy and I miss him. I'm still not sure what a stepfather is, but I know one thing. John was my friend and I'm thankful he was always there for me.

My life was more fun with him in it.

Judy's Speech

Dear John, I'm thinking about love a lot lately. The concept, what it means, what it is in reality, and how we idealize it, how we experience it, how we give it, how we receive it, how we expect it, how we take it for granted, how we ruin it, how we fix it, how we demand it, hoard it, and how we need it. Ultimately, it's different for all of us. But here's what I know.

There is that love you experience as a newborn. Hopefully, it's secure, reliable, soft, nurturing, life-sustaining. Mothering. Fathering. Family-ing. Prepping. Launching.

There is the awakening, the growing, the seeing the world with naive eyes, a wonderful kind of love. It's sensory. It's overwhelming. It's silent. It's loud. It's chaos. It's light, grey and colorful. It's blinding. Light-hearted. Heavy. Uncertain. Informative. Expansive.

There is the crush. The hormonal, oxytocin-inducing, brain-fogging, exhilarating, ridiculous but oh so serious first love. Giving us a taste of what is to come as we mature and hopefully make wise decisions in the presence of intoxicating procreating chemicals when we choose a lover, a partner, a forever friend.

A sunrise, a wave in the ocean, a newborn foal seeking solace from its mare. A tornado. The Cubs winning the series. A straight flush. A prairie dog popping up from a desert mound. Fresh powder. A BBQ. A walk in the Marina. A toast to the Warriors. A perfectly set table. A spilled glass of red wine. Tahoe. Do we take life for granted? Sometimes. Yet we celebrate. And we forget. We regret. Imperfection. It is all Love.

There is John. There is Erica. There is John and Erica. One word. A unit made better by the parts fitting together just so. A thousand-piece puzzle that was started forty-one years ago. It almost didn't happen. But it had to. And so, piece by piece. Still individuals but combining into something much more. We all got to witness you together. The intimacy. The intensity. The humor. Endurance. Your head shaking "I give" in a smile as you surrender in a silly marital spat.

Together, your home was open to us all. It was our home. Each of us is a witness to your love. Our family felt it. Friends saw it. Oh my. That is love. John, you are home to all of us.

I see your reddish, now grayish oh so Scottish hair and dappled skin and mischievous twinkle in your eyes. Your smile that escorts an outsized, full body giggle, the Uncle John Beard giggle. Irresistible. Comforting. Warm. Accepting. It's love.

You love my sister as no one could. You get her. You get all of us. You're the reluctant extrovert. The magnetic center of attention who can't wait for everyone to go home. But no one will ever really know that about you. Because you love.

You're the belly we all want to embrace us. Be hugged by. How Erica pestered you to lose the beautiful soft dad bod belly. I'm so glad you didn't. We all need it, our security blanket, our lazy boy perfect cat bed John chair of reassurance, comfort and love.

You told me over three years ago. "Judy, I'm worried about my brain. I'm not remembering so well. I think something is wrong." There is always the impulse to minimize it, to call it "normal aging". To give false reassurance. I saw the worry in your eyes. I acknowledged your fear. I know too well by now that often when people fear something is amiss, I take it as real. People know themselves. Their bodies. Their intuition. You told me then, if "it" happens, that you don't want to ride the usual course of this wretched disease.

I try to look at all the beauty around me and there is oh so much beauty. It's flattened a bit because I know I have to say my good-bye. We are all saying our good-bye, and no one wants to. No one ever wants to. We all have our individual relationships with you, John. Each one is so precious, so meaningful and unique. So much love.

Is this why love is so beautiful, and so simple at its core? Because we all know that we have to leave.

I do not want you to go. I want you here forever. But more than I don't want you to leave, I don't want you to stay for the wretched, unfair demise that this fucked-up cruel disease inflicts. You are too good for that.

I have to practice my beliefs now. I have been praying for the end of your suffering. I want your suffering to end. I want you to stay. Ultimately, that is how I see love. We all have to loosen our grip. It's a clinging that we have released. Because that is not love. Let the one who is in pain go. Let our love be big enough, unselfish enough, wise enough, courageous enough, to tolerate the grief that will come. Because that is what grief is. Love with nowhere to go.

I am filled with tears of sadness, of relief for you, of joy that my sister brought your giant oversized heart into our fold. Another brother. We needed more brothers.

Now, I wish you rest. I wish you relief from this curse of a disease. I wish for your suffering to end. I wish you courage. I wish you peace. You have my love, forever and ever and ever.

XOXOXO Jude.

A Promise Kept

Lauren's Speech

Oh, my dearest Uncle John, As I sit here struggling to put words to all of the profound feelings of love and admiration I have for you, I feel that I'm bound to fall short because there are just no words to express the immeasurable gratitude each and every one of us has for the joy and laughter that you have filled our lives with, and that you will continue to do each time we think of you.

You may not know it, but you have been such a consistent source of strength and grounding for me in my life. Even during the times where I've really struggled (and let's be honest here: I'm still a ways away from having my shit together) I have felt nothing but complete understanding and compassion from you. I know you have been through so much in your life, probably things beyond my imagination, but they have brought you to be the beautiful, kind person that you are. You truly are a self-made man and the confidence and joy you radiate is tangible and contagious to everyone that crosses your path. We always described you as the kind of guy that goes into a movie theater and comes out with five new friends, and for all of this I look up to you SO. MUCH.

This is the same spirit that my dad had and it has been such a familiar comfort to see it in you too ever since he's been gone. I will do my very best to carry this kind of spirit and attitude of lightness with me too. The way I see it, only the strongest souls out there go through the heaviest burdens and come out of it with a demeanor of lightness. And that's how I've always felt about you- I may walk up the steps to 2219 North Point in my head and with a heavy heart, but as soon as I open the door and hear your voices, I feel a calmness, a sense of acceptance, at ease with and suddenly able to laugh at life. I have so much respect for you as a person and I'm so grateful for your ginormous presence in our family.

You have brought me so much joy both as a kid and as an adult, and once I start reminiscing, the memories just keep rolling… earthquake, John Beard, Johnny Rockets, sneaking me quarters on the pier…but above it all I just hear the echo of that full laughter of yours, a laughter that's filled with wisdom, heart, warmth, and love.

When you have to go, please know it's okay. Because you are leaving us all with a lifetime of that warmth and those smiles each and every time we think of you.

And if you're gonna be watchin' over me, do me a favor and keep that good sense of humor when I fuck up!!

I love you now, tomorrow, forever.

Laurie Loo

Frank's Speech

I'd like to begin with a poem, written 138 A.D., by the Roman Emperor, Hadrian, in his final hours.

Dear, little wandering lovely soul,

the guest and companion of my body,

into what regions will you now depart,

you pale little thing, naked and stiff,

A Promise Kept

unable to crack jokes as usual.

Unable to crack jokes as usual. You can easily imagine John laughing at that line. And what a great laugh it was, too. There is no better testimony to the worth of an individual than the people who come to acknowledge and celebrate their life and passing. But this gathering isn't for John, although I'm sure he would enjoy it. It's for all of us. To that end, I'd like to offer some thoughts that hopefully will make his loss a little more bearable.

What makes life important?

First of all, John wasn't a stuffy formal guy, and he wasn't much for gated communities, so I hope he wasn't too disappointed when he got to heaven… I hear they have gates, but I don't know for sure. But I do know that if those gates squeak or are a little out of true, John will have a remedy. Because he knew how to do stuff. And he wanted you to know what he knew and that made for some interesting and far-ranging conversations.

That's something that makes life important. Because life is for learning, which is fed by *curiosity*, something John had in spades. Nobody arrives here with an owner's manual, and there's a heck of a lot of stuff they don't put in the brochure. John not only knew how to do things, he used his curiosity to figure out things he didn't know and he took a great deal of pleasure and pride in that, and rightly so.

Take those tomatoes he'd grow in that little greenhouse of his. If some satellites were whizzing by over San Francisco and made a heat map photo of the city, that little rectangle would have lit up like a neon sign. I've taken showers that weren't as humid as that little thing.

Erica Baccus

You have brought me so much joy both as a kid and as an adult, and once I start reminiscing, the memories just keep rolling… earthquake, John Beard, Johnny Rockets, sneaking me quarters on the pier…but above it all I just hear the echo of that full laughter of yours, a laughter that's filled with wisdom, heart, warmth, and love.

When you have to go, please know it's okay. Because you are leaving us all with a lifetime of that warmth and those smiles each and every time we think of you.

And if you're gonna be watchin' over me, do me a favor and keep that good sense of humor when I fuck up!!

I love you now, tomorrow, forever.

Laurie Loo

Frank's Speech

I'd like to begin with a poem, written 138 A.D., by the Roman Emperor, Hadrian, in his final hours.

> *Dear, little wandering lovely soul,*
>
> *the guest and companion of my body,*
>
> *into what regions will you now depart,*
>
> *you pale little thing, naked and stiff,*

A Promise Kept

unable to crack jokes as usual.

Unable to crack jokes as usual. You can easily imagine John laughing at that line. And what a great laugh it was, too. There is no better testimony to the worth of an individual than the people who come to acknowledge and celebrate their life and passing. But this gathering isn't for John, although I'm sure he would enjoy it. It's for all of us. To that end, I'd like to offer some thoughts that hopefully will make his loss a little more bearable.

What makes life important?

First of all, John wasn't a stuffy formal guy, and he wasn't much for gated communities, so I hope he wasn't too disappointed when he got to heaven... I hear they have gates, but I don't know for sure. But I do know that if those gates squeak or are a little out of true, John will have a remedy. Because he knew how to do stuff. And he wanted you to know what he knew and that made for some interesting and far-ranging conversations.

That's something that makes life important. Because life is for learning, which is fed by *curiosity*, something John had in spades. Nobody arrives here with an owner's manual, and there's a heck of a lot of stuff they don't put in the brochure. John not only knew how to do things, he used his curiosity to figure out things he didn't know and he took a great deal of pleasure and pride in that, and rightly so.

Take those tomatoes he'd grow in that little greenhouse of his. If some satellites were whizzing by over San Francisco and made a heat map photo of the city, that little rectangle would have lit up like a neon sign. I've taken showers that weren't as humid as that little thing.

And he figured it all out, how to grow tomatoes in cold, foggy San Francisco, complete with that catchment watering system, as reliable as a Roman aqueduct and just as ingenious. I remember the day he showed it to me, as proud of it as you could be over an inanimate object. He described how the whole thing worked, how he had watched the rain run off his neighbor's roof, and how he figured he could capture it and send it down through this Willy-Wonka-type system of pipes and storage tanks that essentially provided him with free water practically all year long.

And how about that train set he built attached to the ceiling in the garage? Even the underside of that thing was beautiful, like a giant integrated circuit board. But that was John, taking that creative spark, that gift from the gods and turning it into anything, an elaborate kid's toy, an irrigation system, a summer's worth of absolutely perfect hot house-grown tomatoes. I like to imagine the satisfaction he got from all of it, that, and just as importantly, the joy he shared with the rest of us as a result.

That leads me to something else that makes life important: *authenticity*. They say you should always be yourself because everyone else is taken. And John really understood that. He knew who he was, he knew what was important to him, and he followed his instincts, his inner voice, with care and conviction. And once he made his mind up to do something, no matter how crazy it may have seemed at the time, he was committed to his choice. And that made it the right thing to do because he was always true to himself. He was, quite simply, one of the most clear-headed individuals I've ever known. Erica recently told me a story about this. Quite a few years ago, John came home from work one day and announced that he had quit his job. Erica was like, "You what?! What are you going to do!" John replied that he was going to take care of their grandkids—Gretchen was about to give birth—but coincident with that, she would also be diagnosed with cancer. And John was there, at the exact right place and right time, right where he was supposed to be, where he was needed most. That was certainly lucky and maybe nothing more than a coincidence, but there was also an awful lot of intention in it, and as I'm sure John knew, living with intention is how you make your own luck. And that's because Intention is something else that makes life important.

We're all going to leave this life at some point. The difference between John and the rest of us is that he knew when that was going to happen. And I thought quite a bit about what it must have been like for him in those last few months, knowing that whatever it was he was doing, he was likely doing for the very last time. Think about that. Most of the time, we sleepwalk through our lives, distracted, distraught, over something that we won't remember 5 minutes later. But John must have been fully engaged, fully present with every fiber of his being, whether he was talking to a child he'd helped raise, holding the woman he loved and shared his life with, or enjoying the taste of tomato he'd grown. What a gift. Not just in the form of the memories he left behind with the people he loved and spent those moments with, but for himself, too. To experience life in that way, in all its exquisite joy and pain, full on, without reservation. What a way to go. We should be so lucky to experience that awareness, that presence, that intention, in our own lives. The ancient Greeks contended that you should call no man happy until he was dead. They understood that, then as now, life will throw things at you that will knock you down and you won't even see them coming. John had one of those things happen to him. But I saw him back in April, and you never would have known it. We spent time together as friends and we laughed together as we always did. I have that as my last memory of him and I think that's how he wanted it. And even though he knew his time was short, he was happy. Why? Because he was grateful for the life he had.

Buddhist monks, scientists and philosophers who study the subject of happiness agree that *gratitude* is the one thing that separates happy people from unhappy people. Most people expect happiness to descend on them when they've ticked off everything on their to-do lists, gotten that big promotion or when things are in general finally all hunky-dory. It doesn't work that way. You have to be grateful for all of it. The joy and the pain, the sweetness and the stonk, because one does not exist without the other. John knew that, too.

One of the most profound ideas I've ever heard about death came from an episode of the now-20-year old tv series, Six Feet Under. In one particular episode, a grieving relative asks one of the young undertakers, "Why do people have to die?" And he answers simply, "so life will be important." You see, if life just went on and on and on, without the possibility of ever losing it, or of there never being an ending of some kind, what value would it have? The very fact that it's finite, that our lives can and will cease to exist for reasons both sublime and ridiculous, at any moment, is what makes life precious.

John understood this because in a very real way, death was not a theoretical construct for him. He could see it right in front of him. And, he bravely chose to embrace it. So, it turns out that, ironically enough, as if there weren't enough irony in life, that death is what makes life important.

Still with me? Okay, home stretch here.

I'd be remiss if I didn't mention John's golf game. John and I played a lot of golf together, not so much these last few years, but at one point, we decided we were actually going to practice and we were going to get better. And we did, but the new reality of our new-found skill becoming more important didn't sit all that well with us. We were like two cavemen who'd accidentally discovered fire. It was like, Whoa, what do we do now? Shortly after that we slipped back to being the hackers we'd always been.

I don't think he really cared. And that was one of the reasons he was so much fun to play with. No matter how good or bad we played, we always enjoyed it. And I think the ability to do that is something else that makes life important. Life is difficult. But you better find a way to enjoy it because it's a long time to be miserable.

And it's funny, but golf is a lot like life and the game is kind of a personality test. You can learn more about a person in four hours on the golf course than you can in four years of marriage counseling. Trust me on that.

John wasn't fun to play golf with because he was a good golfer. He was fun to play with because he was a good friend and a good man leading a good life. And that brings me to the last thing that makes life important.

Goodness.

The philosopher Margaret Nussbaum put it this way:

The condition of being good is that it should always be possible for you to be morally destroyed by something you couldn't prevent. To be a good human being is to have a kind of openness to the world, an ability to trust uncertain things beyond your own control, that can lead you to be shattered in very extreme circumstances for which you were not to blame. That says something very important about the human condition of the ethical life: that it is based on a trust in the uncertain and on a willingness to be exposed; it's based on being more like a plant than like a jewel, something rather fragile, but whose very particular beauty is inseparable from its fragility.

The reason we're all here and feel sad at John's passing is directly related to his goodness. People who are evil creeps are immune from tragedy, and, when something bad does befall them, no one sheds a tear. Couldn't care less. Because it's goodness and its manifestation in another that makes life worth living, and worth having. Goodness makes things like love, kindness, joy, friendship, honor, integrity, trust, happiness, and so much more possible. Unfortunately, goodness is also the one thing that makes tragedy possible.

So, I'll leave you with one last story that reminded me of John. It's from the 13th century Islamic poet, Rumi.

A man in prison is sent a prayer rug by his friend. What he had wanted, of course, was a file, or a crowbar, or better yet, a key! But he began using the rug, praying five-times a day, before dawn, at noon, at mid-afternoon, after sunset and before sleep, as is the custom. And as he used the rug, bowing, sitting up, bowing again, he noticed an odd pattern in the weave of the rug, just at the qilba, as it's called, the place where his head touches. He studies and meditates on that pattern, and he gradually realizes that it is a diagram of the lock that confines him in his cell, and it shows how it works. This is how he is able to escape.

John found himself in prison, too. And it was everything he was, his soul and his spirit — his authenticity, his curiosity, his gratitude, his humor, his goodness, and yes, even his willingness to accept the tragedy of his death, that led him, in the end, to discover his freedom.

Acknowledgements

I have so many people to thank for helping me bring this story to life. First, I must express my gratitude to Alison Luterman who instructed me in her writing class. It was my first ever. When I shared a few pieces of writing with her, she said, "Erica, you have a book here." She encouraged me to continue writing and helped me see I had a story to tell.

Allison Landa became my writing coach and now has the formal title of editor. What would I do without her? Allison first said to me, "You need a scene here, Erica." I asked, "What's a scene?" That is where I started and thanks to Allison whom I now call friend, I have written a book. Most importantly, though, she knew how to push me to think deeper to acknowledge my feelings.

Anne Hamilton, a dear friend, Hollywood writer and director, read early chapters for me. She provided me with no-nonsense feedback challenging me to go inside and find the emotional moments. She taught me that readers want to feel and get to know the real people in the story. Thanks to Anne my writing went from plot to important themes.

Thank you to Deepika Sandhu, publisher of *Soul Sparks Press*, who believed in me from the beginning and became my cheerleader, marketing guru, and inspired me to keep on writing. She is not only my publisher, but my marketer and publicist. As a first time author, the attention and education she has given me is much valued. Her energy, enthusiasm and empathy are contagious and appreciated. She is an inspiration to be admired.

A Promise Kept

Thank you, Dan, Judy, and Keith, for being by my side throughout this journey with John and supporting me through all my tears and grief. Even as words are supposed to flow from me, I do not have enough of them to express my gratitude for their love and kindness.

I also wish to thank Dignitas for the gift they gave John.

If I haven't said it enough, I shall say it again.

Thank you, dear John, for the joy and love
you shared with me for forty-one years.

A Message from John

www.ingramcontent.com/pod-product-compliance
Lightning Source LLC
Chambersburg PA
CBHW050525100526
44581CB00007B/135/J